Accidental Martyr

Survival Guide
For
Family Caregivers
Of Dementia

Kim Joanne Holden
www.kimjoanneholden.com

DEDICATION

This book is dedicated to all Family Caregivers of
Dementia wherever you are.

You are the Unsung Heroes.

I especially dedicate this book to my Mom.
Whom I dearly love and truly miss.

ACKNOWLEDGMENT

For All the Encouragement,

Understanding and Support

I received from Family and Friends

Especially

My Dad and my Uncle

With

Special thanks

to

Victoria

www.kimjoanneholden.com

TABLE OF CONTENTS

JUST FOR YOU

That's right. First and foremost, this book is for YOU the FAMILY CAREGIVER. It's about what you need to know and/or do to prevent caregiver abuse and burnout while caring for someone with dementia. Think of it as your survival guide. A buffet of workable solutions.

With each story, I share the dilemma I experienced, how I handled it and what I learned. At the end of each chapter I list 'Lessons Learned' which you can choose to use or ignore.

We hear a lot about senior abuse, and rightly so. But what about family caregiver abuse? Let's give family caregiver abuse the same attention and support as we do for seniors.

When we are caregiving we begin thinking 'what's wrong with me'. Believe me, it's not you. The problem is dementia and you're at the receiving end.

In the initial stages of dementia, it's difficult to separate the disease from your relative. Why? Because their personality is still there but dementia pops in and out. You never know what's coming at you.

Very little is written or said about how it will impact you, the caregiver. Unfortunately, I had to create solutions on the 'fly' for 18 months.

I kept turning for answers and getting very little advice, if any at all. There was no guide book. I figured others must be having the same difficulties that I experienced, so I decided to pull my journal together into a book.

Under the weight of caregiving 24/7, the last thing I wanted to read about was the medical effects of Alzheimer's. Outlining what it is and what it does to the person. I was already in the war zone. I was living it. I was in the trenches and I had had enough. I was now in survival mode and in serious need of guidance. Tell me how to cope with the abuse I am experiencing right now!

What I realized was, unless you've experienced the nightmare of family caregiving for someone with dementia, an outsider really has no idea of what the caregiver is experiencing.

And that can be a problem with family. They don't see what the problem is really. They'll say "just ignore it", "forget about it"; and my personal favorite, "why take it so personal?' They mean well. It reminds me of the saying, 'the road to hell is paved with good intentions'.

We need support, understanding and compassion. Caring for our loved one is personal. And the abuse we receive is even more so than anyone could believe.

Family Caregivers are in unchartered waters. This book, I hope will change that.

You really are performing a wonderful, self-sacrificing service.

I hope this book helps you smile, laugh and realize you are not alone.

You are Truly Awesome!

MOM & AL

In my case, I realized what I was experiencing was not my mom as I knew her. Although it sounds like mom, looks likes mom and uses the 'I'm your mother" card. It's only about 60% mom (my guess). Alzheimer's has taken squatters rights on the rest.

I love my mother. We have always had a very close relationship. But I was noticing I was beginning to dislike my mom very much and I didn't like that feeling. So I analyzed the situation realizing it was what Alzheimer's was doing to my mom that I hated. So I came up with a solution. Whenever I had to deal with her Alzheimer symptoms, I referred to it simply as 'Mom & AL' – 'AL' is short for Alzheimer's.

LESSON LEARNED:

When you realize you're resenting the abusive treatment you're receiving, create a "Mom & AL" term in order to separate your negative feelings from your relative and the disease.   Mom & AL. Dad & AL. You get the idea!

Unfortunately, they don't have any filters now that stop them from saying or doing what is an inappropriate behavior or comment. Sad to say, that part of your loved one is gone.

MAC TRUCK
HEADING YOUR WAY

Y ou will feel like a Mac Truck has run you over by
the time caregiving has taken its toll on you. It is
how I referred to the state I felt I was in whenever
anyone asked me how I was doing.

By taking care of your relative with dementia (mother
in my case), and possibly you are also the assigned Power of
Attorney, **in the diseased mind of your loved one you
are**:

- …the **Evil Child**. Or the worst sibling ever
(assuming there is another) or just the worst person
imaginable. Even as you do everything for them,
everyone else, especially those who don't visit often,
are fantastic; but not you.

- ...**a Thief**. You are stealing from them on every level imaginable (i.e. money, property, cottages, houses, vehicle, papers, clothes, food, bed linen, laundry, photographs, diaries, ornaments, plants and more). If they can think of it, you are stealing it. Other people might be accused of stealing from them too, but you're the absolute worst person they have the misfortune to know, or have given birth to. There's nothing that will change their mind. So you'll just have to get used to it.

- ...**the Enemy**, as told to me by a lawyer

- ...**the Ugly Reminder** that they have dementia. They are losing their independence and their mind. Understandably, they don't like it. They will blame someone because it's not their fault. (Not that fault enters into it.) You're the closest person to them and they're relying heavily on you. Lucky you! You get to feel their frustration and anger because you're in their face every day

You are also now **experiencing Caregiving Abuse**, such as:

- ...**Lies about you** are told to anyone who will listen about how you're taken advantage of them (i.e. stealing listed above). They are adamant about what they are saying and are totally believable. Mom & AL look normal, sound normal. How is anyone to know that what Mom & AL are saying is coming from a diseased mind?

- …Being on the receiving end of their **verbal attacks** on you personally that are just downright nasty. They know which buttons to push (after all they probably raised you and helped create those buttons!) and they push every one of them as hard as they can. They hold that button down for as long as their strength will allow them. And if you cry or show any weakness? They'll push some more! It's power. It's spiteful. And Mom & AL *love* it.

- …**Character Assassination and Bullying** 24/7 from someone you love, and you thought loved you. You're now a victim. It's daily abuse thrown at you. I realized there were no filters with Dementia. If they can think it, they will say it. Unfortunately for you, they never seem to think happy thoughts! Oh, how I wish they would!

- …**You "Don't Do Anything"** for them. This is my favorite. Even though *you do everything* for them. Such as book and take them to all medical appointments, sit with them in the Emergency Room for 8 hours at a time, do their shopping, house cleaning, maintenance repairs, food preparation, laundry, banking, pay all their bills, assist them when they need help and/or get confused, handle all problems on their behalf, get woken up by them throughout the night, nurse them when they're sick and so much more. All this of course, is done without any monetary compensation. This is not a paid occupation. You're happy to help them but a thank-you would be nice. Think again. With Mom & AL at the wheel, thanks isn't happening.

And then you will begin to think:

- …Am I losing my mind?

- …What's wrong with me?

- …Am I developing dementia too? I can't remember like I used to

- …What the hell's going on?

- …What have I done to deserve this?

- …Am I as bad as he/she says I am?

- …Is it just me? Am I the only one experiencing this?

- …Who has he/she told all those lies to?

- …OMG, what am I going to do if people believe those lies? How do I stop it?

- …I'm doing my best to care for her/him and she/he treats me this way!? Seriously?

And you will begin to feel:

- …Confused, betrayed, maligned and possibly alone, but definitely unappreciated

And then you will be:

- …Suffering sleep deprivation

- …Stress induced illnesses

- …Emotionally and physically exhausted so much so that you have to take prescribed medications to handle your responsibilities

- …Final diagnosis will be about you, not Mom & AL, because now you've suffering with Caregiver Burnout

- …And who's going to take care of You?

Does this sound like you? Do you relate to any of the above? No doubt you do.

Don't worry. You're doing what you were asked to do, as caregiver or Power of Attorney. You were chosen to act on their behalf when the time came that they could not. You were chosen to do the job because they trusted your decisions. They knew you would respect their wishes.

Nobody knew (not even our loved one) that 'Mom & AL' would be driving a Mac Truck heading straight for you! So if we don't know what's coming, how could anyone be prepared for it? There's a lot of information about Elder Abuse and rightly so.

But this book is about *HELPING YOU* protect yourself from Dementia Abuse and Caregiver Burnout.

And so my story begins…..

SOMETHING'S
SERIOUSLY WRONG

Visiting mom was no longer enjoyable. She was verbally abusive about my appearance, apparent inability to get a boyfriend (she assures me wearing Shalimar perfume does the trick) and just being a lousy daughter.

My mother and I have always been very close since my dad died when I was 4 years old. We knew each other's secrets and always confided in each other. I knew something was now seriously wrong but I couldn't put my finger on it

It got so bizarre, I would only now visit mom with another person present, usually Vivian who I've known since we were 10 years old, so she knew mom well. I was living in Toronto at the time, and would pick Vivian up enroute and drive out to visit mom an hour away. Mom still got nasty with me but it was contained. I asked Vivian if I was imaging it. No, she was puzzled too.

Another mutual friend, Sandy, was noticing a change in mom too. Sandy would correct mom when mom was badmouthing me, because what she was saying just wasn't true. Mom would argue with her that she was right.

On one occasion mom even kicked Sandy out of her apartment because Sandy was defending me to my mom! Mom had actually accused me of stealing some papers which Sandy eventually found in mom's apartment.

It's a blessing having a mutual friend in your court. Sandy told me of conversations mom had with her that were derogatory towards me. It was a heads-up for me. What the heck was going on?

THE CAR

Mom offered me her old pristine Volvo, as she had just purchased another car, which was unusual because she loved her Volvo. My car had broken down on the Don Valley Parkway in Toronto returning from work one hot summer's day. A friend had rescued me from the highway and loaned me his leased business vehicle.

So when mom offered her Volvo to me - that was a real blessing. Good news, I told my friend! His lease was up and it had to be returned. Perfect timing.

Mom also received an unsolicited offer of $1500 to purchase her Volvo. She withdrew her offer when mom told her she was giving me the car.

Guess what? Mom's decided to sell the Volvo to a man who had recently befriended her at his place of work, a retail store. Originally the price for him to buy the Volvo was $800, and then later he got her down to $500. After all, there was a small crack in the windshield he said.

In explaining her change of mind to me, she said with my contract job she felt I couldn't repair the Volvo if needed, so she decided to sell it to her new retail friend. Because she gave her 'word' to this guy, she would not sell it to Sandy either who has helped mom so much over the years, nor give it to me. Nothing made sense.

At this time I was temporarily living with mom. So one evening I came home from work to find mom's apartment disheveled. She was frantic. Her retail friend had given her the $800 all in 20's. She put it in her special box and now it was empty. I checked the apartment; no monies to be found.

She didn't sleep that night. She got me up early in the morning, tripped and fell onto the hardwood floor. I laid her on the couch with some ice.

During this time, she gave me her retail friends' cell phone number to call him to verify he had given her the monies. In mom's presence, on the phone I asked him if any money passed hands and he said 'no' because there was a crack in the windshield and he had to think about it. Mom was sitting 3 feet away from me. She heard every word spoken, as I held the phone away from my ear with the volume up loud. He lied. When it comes to money, mom has a *really* good memory. If there were $800 worth of 20's in her hand, damn sure she'd remember that.

My guess is that he changed his mind, saw where mom put the cash and retrieved it without telling her when she got him a beverage.

I stayed with mom for the morning, putting ice on her head, made her breakfast and off to work I went. I was relieved to see that her Volvo was still in the underground parking lot. So at least there was no problem in the long run.

Although I called in that I would be late for work, my boss wasn't happy with me.

I came home to find mom perturbed once again. Her retail friend had called her back after I went to work. He said he wouldn't visit her while I was living there. He said I had attitude! The real shocker was that my mom totally sided with him! After telling me off, she sent me to my room!

I couldn't believe it. My mom didn't stand up for me when I'm doing something *she's asked me* to do!!!!! What was going on?

(He soon got the car though. I later found the hand written receipt of $500 for the Volvo. This "decent guy" (that's what mom called him) who dickered down the price of her car to $500. The real bonus was he also got her tool box filled with jewelry she kept in her trunk. That red tool box has never been seen since. He's never called her again either.)

I went to visit my brother Steven at 11pm that night. He was a musician so I knew he'd be up late. We had tea and I told him what was going on. It was just crazy. He knew something just wasn't quite right with mom, but we couldn't put our finger on it.

LESSONS LEARNED:

Mom's 'don't tell me what to do' speech was her normal, but it meant now she wasn't reasoning on anything her friends or family was saying. She was throwing caution out the window. More defiant than normal.

She already had a good working car (Volvo) she was proud of in excellent working order. She goes out and purchases a used vehicle on the spur of the moment and it wasn't even the type of car she had always admired.

She was also waiting to do her driving test to see if she would qualify to renew her driver's license as she was in her 80's. Timing was all wrong. The vehicle type was wrong. The car sale price was really wrong. It was still mom, but the dementia signs were blaring. She was now showing signs of not making sound decisions. But there was no stopping her.

So pay attention to the red flags you'll be witnessing. It's the beginning of many more to come. You'll know it. It just won't feel right or make any sense.

The difficulty is that at this stage, their behavior flips in and out of dementia. That's where the confusion begins for us. And whatever decision or comment they make, they are adamant they are right. You can't challenge their decision because they won't reason with you.

You cannot exercise Power of Attorney until they have been assessed by an expert that they are incapable.

So if their behavior raises a question in your mind, realize it's Mom & AL taking control. If you are thinking "what's he/she doing?" It's Mom & AL. If it puzzles you, then it's Mom & AL. These are the red flags signaling dementia.

IN THE BEGINNING
...There Were Police

The park is almost vacant. It's almost 3:30 in the afternoon. Squirrels are bouncing about. The waves of Lake Ontario are greyish and cold. I wanted to sit at the picnic table, drink my coffee and listen to the waves hit the shore. But it's just too darn cold! So, sit in the car it is.

There's an elderly couple in the distance walking along the boardwalk. She's slowly using her walker and he's patiently walking slowly beside her. I relate to what I'm seeing, and turn my attention away because I just can't watch it. Gees, I can't believe I'm enjoying watching squirrels collect nuts! Oh my goodness, what's happening to me? Am I losing my mind? Feels like it!!

Nine months ago, I moved in with my mom who now has Moderate Dementia. She has short-term memory loss diagnosed with Alzheimer's and Mixed Vascular Dementia.

I have seen the good, the bad and the ugly. What an unimaginable learning curve. I know there are thousands of us out there trying to take care of family members with dementia without a 'How-To' manual. It's tough going, to say the least.

For my sanity, I journaled the shenanigan's I was wrestling with. As time progressed I decided to share my experiences and coping strategies. Let's start with a good one.

As was my Saturday custom, I was gone for the day visiting my grandchildren on the other side of the city. Mom felt too tired to come with me and stayed home this particular day.

Later that night, I met up with friends and had a nice evening watching the hockey game at a sports bar. Imagine my surprise when I realized I was in the neighbourhood where my father was raised! (He died when I was 4 years old). I couldn't remember the street name, so I called mom to help me locate the house. Sure, she's got short term memory loss, but not long term. It was a good idea, but she didn't remember the street name. It was now 10 pm and I told her I'd be home in a couple of hours. Not a problem, she said. She had eaten and was enjoying her favorite television shows.

I arrived home at midnight. Opened the door of our apartment and met two young police officers standing by the entrance with my mom sitting on the couch with a smug look on her face. "Tell her off" she said to the officers.

I asked if there was a problem. Before the officers answered, my mom asked me "Was I supposed to know where you were?" I politely reminded her of our weekly Saturday routine of visiting the grandchildren, and that today she was too tired to make the visit, and that I had called her this evening to make sure she was okay.

The officers told me they received a 911 call from my mother stating that her daughter was MISSING! That's ME! I'm a grandmother of three! The officers must have been surprised when mom opened her door to find a woman 83 years old had lost her daughter! Mom said she was trying to remember the names of people I knew, so she could send the officers over to their place to find me!

The officers were very understanding. In their opinion, I appeared old enough to be out at this late hour and decided to leave. Mom was a little, just a little bit embarrassed. We had tea and laughed about it. I appreciated her concern and love. Isn't that what mom's do?

LESSON LEARNED:

Have only one telephone number handy for them (preferably your cell phone) that they can contact you. Have it on speed dial on their phone. Make sure your name is legible for them to read.

This just might stop them from calling everyone you know at a late hour trying to locate you. Remember, with dementia, they're not registering time of day. It's either 12 noon or midnight. If they're up, so is everyone else!

Your friends and family will thank you!

Kim Joanne Holden

ELUSIVE PEPPER SQUASH

J ust got home lugging all my groceries into the kitchen. As my habit, I immediately put everything away.

Now, I would have sworn I bought a pepper squash (a.k.a. acorn squash). I recall seeing it on the conveyor belt at the cash register when checking out of the grocery store. I remember the weight of the bag carrying it into the apartment. It certainly felt like a pepper squash was in the bag. I would have sworn I left it on the kitchen counter, but for the life of me I can't find it! I asked my mom if she had seen the squash. She said she had but had no idea where it was.

Now if you aren't familiar with a pepper squash; it's deep green, heavy, approximately the size and shape of a medium bunch of bananas and not easy to miss! Perhaps I could describe it as a small, dark green pumpkin. I trust you get the picture that this isn't something that gets easily mislaid.

Did it roll under a table? Under a chair? Roll somewhere in the living room? Not that it actually rolls, but quoting Sir Arthur Conan Doyle, "Once you eliminate the impossible, whatever remains, no matter how improbable, must be the truth". What else could have happened to it?

I'm becoming obsessed with finding this elusive pepper squash. I checked the apartment hallway. No pepper squash. Elevator? No pepper squash. I retraced my steps to the underground parking lot. No pepper squash. Checked the car back seat and trunk. No pepper squash. I scanned the apartment carpeted hallway once again to see if perhaps it fell out of my bag. No pepper squash.

Where on earth can this thing be? For anyone watching me, I must have looked like a crazy woman. I'm going to bed retracing my steps trying to remember where I had put it. I swear I had put it on the kitchen counter. After several days trying to find it, I gave up. I guess the only way I'm going to find it is when it rots and I'll follow my nose or the flies, whichever comes first.

It took another 2 days to accidently find this squash. You'll never guess where! I happened to go into the solarium to sweep out the leaves in case any fell off of mom's plants. Lo and behold! There sits my pepper squash! Mom had planted it in one of her earth filled flower pots! I had a good laugh at this. I even took a picture. To this day, I cannot resist smiling whenever I see a pepper squash!

LESSEN LEARNED:

Don't go crazy trying to find something. If Mom & AL had anything to do with it, you won't find it easily.

Give your brain a rest and put the problem aside. Hopefully, you'll stumble upon it as I did!

CHERISH THE GOOD MEMORIES

When I was told mom had early signs of dementia, I read as much as possible on the subject to slow down the disease.

So I bought children's puzzles to do with mom, although she's not a puzzle person. I've read it helps the brain. I chose children's puzzles because the pieces are larger and easier to pick up. With aging, mom's fingers have lost their ridges. Also the larger pieces makes the puzzle quicker to complete. Mom would lose interest if it took over an hour to do.

I may have said before that my mom is an artistic person. What I noticed for the first time was that in working on the puzzle together – I look for shapes, she looks for shades of colors! This was such a nice moment for me. At this age, I learned something new about my mom!

WHO'S ON FIRST?

My mom pokes her head into my room and asks "What's the matter with me? Why do I keep forgetting?" I reply "You have Alzheimer's." "NO, I DON'T HAVE ALZHEIMER'S!" she yells back at me, "And don't ever say that again!" And the she leaves abruptly.

Continuing to work on my laptop, she returns two minutes later poking her head once again into my room. "What's the matter with me? Why do I keep forgetting?" "You have Alzheimer Mom." "NO I DON"T HAVE ALZHEIMER'S and stop saying that!!!"

She wasn't giving up! She just kept coming back over and over again, asking me the same question. Each time she's getting louder and more frustrated. My reply was always the same.

I knew my response had to change or this would go on indefinitely. When she told me to stop saying she had Alzheimer's, I said "okay then, stop asking me what's wrong with you!" And she did!

Kind of reminded me of 'Who's on First' with Abbott and Costello!

THE BIG TIPPER

Mom is famous for never tipping. She grew up on welfare and that is what she learned. "They make more money than I do!" she would always say.

Throughout my life, if I left a tip on the table for the waitress, mom would scoop it up and hand it back to me. I learned to hide my tip under my empty plate or mug so mom wouldn't see it.

Now to the present. Every Monday, the pharmacy delivers mom's prescriptions in a blister pack. Mom comes to me asking for money for a tip! If I don't have any change to give her, she tells the delivery person "my daughter never tips". The first time she said that, my mouth fell open! Once again, mom's having fun with the guy! And I'm laughing in my room!

LESSONS LEARNED:

Cherish these special moments. Record them somehow because you are likely to forget without a reminder. Journal, take a photo or video it. In my experience, the ratio of happy events to sad (angry/frustrating/shocked/abused) is far outweighed, so capture them when you can.

Don't be a martyr. Allow the pharmacy to blister pack all their medications. It helps to track what medications they are/are not taking.

WALKER M.I.A.

Water on in the month, it occurred to me that mom's walker was missing. In our two-bedroom apartment there wasn't many places to hide it. I just couldn't find it.

Mom said she had no idea where the walker was. I checked the apartment hallway. No walker.

I called her brother. He didn't have it. I asked him to double-check his van, just in case. Every Thursday he'd try to take mom to the Adult Day Clinic at the Senior Centre with her walker, so perhaps it was there. Nope, no walker in the van.

When did mom last see it? I got different renditions every time I asked. One was that she just pushed it into the hallway and left it there. Another was that she had called the number on the walker to have it picked up. A man came to the apartment and took the walker with him. Besides, *she* "didn't need a walker". Anyway, she "wouldn't get a boyfriend with one of those things!" I wracked my brain for 7 days. (You'll do this a lot managing Mom & AL). Where could that walker be? It's vanished into thin air. I've called everyone I knew she came in contact with. No one has seen it. I didn't want to give up looking without exhausting all avenues to find it.

Following up on what mom had said, I called the medical supply place where she had purchased the walker a few years ago. They checked all their deliveries within the past week. There was no mention of a walker being picked up. In fact I was told, they would never pick up a walker from a senior who had been prescribed one. It would have been an odd request. (This was probably my first cue that I was dealing with Mom & AL. Live and learn!). Seniors don't stop needing their walker, they told me. They gave me the contact information of mom's occupational therapist in case we needed to reorder the walker.

Impossible to believe, but I had a Deluxe $400 Walker missing in action!

Later that week, by chance, I bumped into our landlady as I was waiting for the elevator from the underground parking garage. I was now desperate. Had she seen mom's walker? Yes! Yahoo! I was doing my happy-dance! Mom gave her the walker stating she didn't need it anymore! Fortunately, she had stored it away.

Joyfully I brought home the walker.

Sadly, I was the only one excited.....

LESSON LEARNED:

If it doesn't feel right, it isn't. If it doesn't make sense, it's because there isn't any. Realize Mom & AL are involved.

Trust your gut. It's *not* you. Stop pulling your hair out because you will go bald!

Mom & AL can be a real pain in the backside! Dementia just goes downhill from here! That's a guarantee!

STRESS SAVERS

This is going to save you a lot of unnecessary stress….Check their pockets!

You think they've taken their pills regularly? They convincingly said they did but their attitude says differently. Check their pockets! It's like a treasure hunt. And when you show them what you found, they'll look at you like they have no idea how they got there. Now the problem is figuring out how long these pills have been hidden. After all, you don't want to double dose them.

I've found pills in the bottom of the washing machine. Pills in housecoat pockets. In fact, anything with pockets is open to possibilities. I've found missing dentures in housecoats, in bed under her pillow, in her dresser drawers, everywhere except in her mouth! She has an older denture which she won't throw away. She'll sometimes wear them

and come to me worried that her gums have shrunk
because the denture doesn't stay up in her mouth!

Dementia creates a hide-and-seek mentality. Mom &
AL does the hiding, and you, the caregiver do the seeking.
Daily you are searching for something they've mislaid.
Mom would hide her purse and then couldn't find it. I'm
searching high and low for it. It could be, and usually is,
anywhere.

One day mom would feel spry and could do her
physical therapy exercises which involves leg raising. The
next day, she couldn't do it. So I videotaped her having
difficulty raising her legs to show the therapist who was
coming the next day. Good thing I did because during this
visit he was going to cancel mom's treatment, believing she
was recovered. He was surprised when I showed him the
recording from the previous day. He felt perhaps it was
because she had just woken up and still too tired to do
them, or possibly she had a brain episode which is most
likely.

LESSONS LEARNED:

Be proactive. If there are pockets, good chance you'll
be surprised what's in them.

Again, filming my mom doing her leg raises at home
(in this case, couldn't do them) allowed the therapist to
have a better understanding of my mom's condition.

It gets to the point you sound unbelievable or in denial when stating something is true, and it's not the case at that moment. Video support is just an easier, indisputable proof of their condition. Save yourself the headaches. Be proactive.

Blister Packs: Get the pharmacy to package all pills in a blister pack. It helps you track what hasn't been taken, and hopefully which time of day.

Plastic Baggies: Collect all pills not taken in something like a Ziploc bag. I did. And took it with us to mom's medical appointment with her family doctor. Why, you may ask? It helps the doctor diagnose and prescribe based on the realization of what mom *isn't* taking in relation to mom's behavior.

If the doctor isn't informed of medications not taken, they will presume that she is taking all medications correctly and might decide to increase the dosage, or prescribe something else. The physician was shocked when I pulled out of my purse a medium size Ziploc bag almost full of drugs my mom refused to take or missed over a 6 month period.

The doctor felt mom's diabetic medication was doing very well because her numbers were excellent. That's when I remembered to show her the bag of unused medications and her eyes widened! So mom had excellent sugar control without medication, and still does. It made an impact to say the least! A picture says a million words, or in my case, a baggie! Sure beats having a discussion about it.

ABNORMAL IS
YOUR NEW NORMAL

It came on sort of all-of-a-sudden, but mom's late night activities has expanded to rearranging things. I'd open the linen closet to find nothing where it was the day before. Open the cutlery drawer in the morning to discover the spoons were missing. She had placed them in a mug and put it on a plate in a cupboard. She would sort through the garbage and put most of it on the kitchen counter in piles.

I'd find her looking for a particular vase that she believed she had hidden money in but couldn't remember which vase. I never knew what I was going to encounter every morning.

Often I would find mom's dirty clothes thrown into her storage cupboard. For about 6 months before I moved in with mom, she adamantly told the story to those who would listen, that someone in the apartment building had stolen her underwear from the laundry room. I would always correct her saying that no one would do that. She was firm in her belief until I found her clean underwear in a bucket stored under papers in her spare room. I know they had been put there wet because mold had grown on them! She was certainly surprised when I found them.

Throughout the night, mom would regularly call for me to fix the television for her. She habitually, but unintentionally pushes the wrong button on the remote and she ends up watching 'snow'. You know, that crackling, fuzzy sound?! Now, you might say I should ignore her and stay in bed. In a perfect world, I would. Unfortunately, besides her continuous calling my name, the sound that now comes from the television is loud and very annoying. I must get up and fix the situation so I can get what little sleep remains.

I have been jolted awake with my mom's face inches away from mine, asking if I was awake!

I'd come home late at night to find my bed stripped of my pillow and comforter. Went into mom's room who smugly told me that I had stolen her linen and she's taken it back. Now my mom missed her calling as an interior decorator. In her house, everything was perfect. So rather than get into an argument (because she looked like she wanted one), I asked her if she would ever buy a king-size comforter for her double bed? She looked over the edge of her bed as my comforter was swimming onto the bedroom

floor. "No, I guess not". She gave me back my comforter
and my pillow. My hand mirror that was standing on her
end table would wait until morning.

Other caregivers have told me similar stories. One
daughter found her mother had stashed hundreds of empty
plastic bags in every drawer of her house. In her dressers,
cupboards, you name it and it contained bags!

On another occasion, I came across a cooked chicken
stored away in my friend's cupboard reserved for plates.
You guessed it! 'Mom & AL' was there too!

LESSONS LEARNED:

What you are experiencing is now your new normal.
It's important for you to realize that you are not alone.
Most caregiver's are going through this too. I would share
my experiences with friends and acquaintances and we'd
end up laughing about it. Find the lighter side. It's healthier
for your mental disposition. It's a form of stress relief.

Try to lessen the work and aggravation for yourself.
Think what their idiosyncrasy is, in my case, garbage
sorting, and remove it! I was diligent in putting out the
trash, otherwise I'd wake up with trash sorted everywhere.
Think of Mom & AL as a child and put things away or out
of reach. There's a saying "out of sight, out of mind". Some
things you can't do anything about, but if you can, do it.

CAREGIVER SUPPORT

Mom had gotten her flu shot but she still got sick. Fortunately for her it was the 24 hour kind. Unfortunately for me, Mom was sick on her bed. And in the garbage can. You know the drill. I was holding her up, walking her to the bathroom. Cleaning her up afterwards. Changing sheets. Okay, you do what you have to do, no problem. The next day she was eating and drinking. She's much better.

I was relieved. She was only sick for one day. I think the flu shot reduced the severity of how sick she could have gotten. I'm not a health professional but I feel strongly about this because, I then got sick! I did not get the flu shot and I was sick much worse than mom was and for much longer.

So here I am hugging the toilet bowl and mom keeps trying to come in to help me. I'm telling her to stay away from me because I didn't want her to get sick again. I had my own problems! She just kept coming into the bathroom over and over again. I'm being sick and she's trying to have a conversation with me! She's offering me food and tea. The more I refused, the more she tried to find something else to give me. It was a mother caring for her little child. Upon reflection it's sweet. At the time, it was really annoying. Now, no one knew either of us had gotten ill. Everyone knew I was taking care of mom. But who was taking care of me?

It's important that family and friends know what you're experiencing. Most of the time, I didn't want to relate the situations over the phone. Just feels like I'm reliving it all over again, and I don't want to. (In fact, it's one reason why it took me several years to put this book together). I type very quickly, so I would email my uncle updates regularly.

So this is a sample of one of my emails I sent to my uncle, mom's brother. He appreciated the updates.

"I came home yesterday at 9pm and found mom lying on the floor. I warmed her up with a heating pad in her bed. She slept well. This morning she had difficulty raising herself off the couch. Fed her porridge and everything seemed as usual.

I've left messages for a few nursing homes to get financial information so I'm prepared when the time comes.

Anyway, later she comes into my room with that familiar 'Alzheimer' perturbed attitude. So apparently she thinks she's living in one of her previous homes. "What's going on? This is my furniture. Who's the guy working outside my house?" Thinks she was in a mental hospital and wanted to know why I put her there. Also thinks I'm living with someone here in my room. She thinks something's going on. She's seeing shadows on the walls that weren't there before. They were also seen in a different room. She wants to know why she's feeling this way. She threatens to see a doctor and lawyer without me. She angrily pushes my hand away when I help her from falling backwards.

I have an appointment tomorrow at 8:45am to talk to her family MD. I'm going alone. I put her on the phone to you because she wants to complain about me but you weren't home. That's the reason for the message she left. So I called dad and asked him to call mom to let her talk. I cannot bear the emotion of it all any more.

I'm trying not to take it all personally although she gets nasty. It's 'AL' talking, not my mom. So if you're around, please give her a call and just let her talk. This is such an ugly disease. I could do with her talking to someone else who knows her situation rather than me.... I need to catch a break."

As you can see, I'm letting him know what a day with Mom & AL is like. It's a short version of the facts.

LESSONS LEARNED:

I should have had support, a back-up in place *for me*! I got really sick and I had no one to call to take mom away, either for the day or overnight. It's not that no one would help. I just couldn't physically call anyone to ask! Can you discuss with family and friends who would be willing to step in when these emergencies arise?

When mom was sick, that should have been a heads-up for me to call family that I might need help with mom. When you, the caregiver, is really sick that is not the time that you can call around for help.

Family appreciate knowing what's going on. Keep them informed. Emails are a great way to inform them of medical appointments and test results.

You will need your family support while you are caregiving. If they know what is happening they can better help and understand your situation. There are two sides to every story. Make sure they also know your side to what's going on while you care for family. For sure Mom & AL are talking. Be proactive and protect yourself.

Getting friends and family to listen to 'Mom & AL' while they vent is a very practical and helpful break for you.

It's therapeutic writing down your feelings. Just get the emotions off your chest and on to the page. You can always throw it out later.

If possible, get to the gym and punch some bags.

Run. Swim. Do yoga. Meditate. Watch comedies. Do something to get the stress off of you, and you like to do it.

Heaven knows you need it and deserve it!

Be safe and healthy.

HOSPITAL APPOINTMENT

Mom could only make it out the front door of our apartment building when she began to feel too weak to walk any further. Her doctor's appointment, fortunately was just across the street at the hospital. So sitting on the seat of her walker, I pushed her across the driveway to the traffic li**ghts.**

She didn't feel strong enough to walk across the street with the lights so while seated, I had to push her across. Before I knew it, the wheels caught a hole in the pavement and just about over she toppled! It happened as if in slow motion. I can still visualize her holding on to her favorite little blue purse with her lips tight across her teeth.

Fortunately, a gentleman nearby helped me recover mom from tipping over. We were laughing so hard about the looks on each other's face! We quickly got to mom's appointment at the GAIN clinic (which helps keep seniors mobile, safe and in their own residence for as long as possible).

Mom and I respectfully take our seat before the doctor. He asks mom how is she doing. While pointing a finger at me, she replies "Why ask me? I've got Alzheimer's! Ask her!" Mom and I burst out laughing, and cautiously, the doctor joined in laughing as well. It was a good moment.

Now here's the puzzling thing. Mom performs the usual cognitive test where she has to draw a clock, remember 3 words and more. She did well in her score testing, drew the clock (don't know if it's cheating for her because she's an artist) but anyway, she even accurately recalled the 3 words later. I was impressed and perplexed.

Why, you may ask? Two days earlier, we both spent most of the day visiting my daughter and grandchildren. When we left their home and I drove to the end of the small court, mom asked me where were we and where were we going? So why didn't she remember the past 4 hours playing, storytelling, laughing, drinking tea with her great grandkids, when we just said good-bye, but she could remember 3 unrelated words in his office?

I asked the doctor to explain this to me. He said that her last MRI showed narrowing of the arteries which could cause the dementia symptoms to fluctuate in being better or worse. Besides Alzheimer's, she also was diagnosed with Vascular Dementia. This could also explain her fatigue, light headedness and falls. They often coexist especially in older patients.

Glad I asked.

Kim Joanne Holden

WHAT NO ONE TELLS YOU

Get legal advice. Go with questions to ask and be prepared to explain the difficulties you are experiencing. Get a clear understanding of what it really mean when you are Power of Attorney over Finances and Personal Care. Get the facts so you will be performing your POA duties honestly and accurately

Find out who is the Capacity Assessor nearest to you. Get your relative assessed if you think their cognitive ability to make decisions is declining. It's also an excellent thing to do so that their cognitive ability can be testified that they *are* capable of making decisions. It goes both ways and is excellent to have done because you don't know how they are going to change.

Shockingly, I have heard that loved ones have been dropped inside hospital emergency waiting rooms with their health card. What I never knew is that they are *never* turned away. They get a bed.

Now, I don't recommend this of course, but it's another red flag. At first read, you will say to yourself, what a horrible thing for a family member to do! And that's true. But there are two sides to every story. Now I invite you to think of it from the caregiver's perspective for a moment. Is it not awful that the caregiver is driven to that extreme means just to get a bed for their loved one?

As long as you live with someone with Alzheimer's, nothing really improves in receiving outside help for their care. It actually stalls because the system is overwhelmed, and, in my opinion, we are cheap labor. They will not increase weekly hours or send more help for her care as long as you're there.

Basically, with you living and caring for your loved one, a Personal Support Worker (PSW) will help dress and bath them, ensure they take their pills and make a meal for them. God bless Personal Support Workers! They work really hard.

Take advantage of this opportunity. Look at it as a break. Get out! Go relax! Give the PSW your cell phone number so they can call you when they're ready to leave so you can return home. It's a blessing.

In Ontario, Canada at least, it can take up to 6 years to get your relative into a newer, nicer nursing home (depending on where you live and the accommodation you are requesting). So don't wait until there's a crisis. Discuss this with your loved one and family.

Contact the proper authorities and get them on the waiting list. You don't have to take the vacancy when one comes up if it's not needed. You will just be dropped to the bottom of the waiting list. On your choice sheet, you'll have to pick approximately 5 nursing homes in your area that are your choices. Rate them 1st choice to 5th. Your relative must sign if cognitive.

Every time your loved one comes out of hospital (surgeries, falls etc.), they get increased hours at home for the 2-3 weeks by Personal Support Workers from the community health services. Then they are reassessed in a 30 minute interview by a nurse who may never have met your loved one before. Have your concerns and questions written out for the nurse so you don't forget anything. Also invite family members to join the meeting. Remember you're stressed out; non-caregiving family members are not. They also have a fresh perspective that you might be missing. Welcome their opinions.

LESSON LEARNED:

NEVER be 'dolled up' during this interview (or any other meeting where a decision will be made). This is not the time to get your hair done, remove facial hair or get dressed up!

If you look like you're coping, you're loved can stay with you. Community health services can only judge the situation on the outside. It's up to YOU to tell them if you can't handle it any more. Don't hold back. If you need to cry; cry. Tell it and show it like it is without any pretense. I've been told to look your worst when you are interviewed by a case worker. It's not what you say; *it's how you say it and how you look*. If you're not getting sleep, your appearance should reflect that.

During the assessment, if you look like you're handling the caregiving well, there is no need to change your loved one's circumstances, regardless of what you say. The case worker might even decrease your loved one's hours of personal support care if you live there. You are not being deceitful. So tell it like it is. If you can't cope, you had better look like it.

If your loved one lived alone, they'd be in a nursing home sooner. Weigh the consequences seriously before caring for them 24/7. If you move in, they are no longer in a crisis because you're there.

POA (Power of Attorney) trumps everything. So if your name is on bank accounts jointly, you are beneficiary, and have signing authority, everything is fine until you must act as Power of Attorney over the finances. Then you have a Conflict of Interest if you are accessing the funds for anything other than your loved one's needs, even if it's previously agreed upon.

Mom's lawyer advised her not to sign anything from the bank relating to POA. Be careful. Banks can make yours and your loved one's life a living nightmare. The lawyers' POA covers everything necessary. Banks have another agenda. Be cautious. Never sign any documents without your lawyers consent. Lawyers are acting in your loved one's best interests; I can't say the same for banks.

Hire a **Certified Capacity Assessor** to assess your loved one, as I mentioned above. Certainly money well spent. Best advice that I followed through on by a lawyer. If the lawyer hadn't told me about this expertise, I would never have known about it.

So what's a Capacity Assessor? They assess whether or not your loved one is capable of making decisions, handle their finances, and take care of themselves et cetera. The Capacity Assessor decision stands up in court. When the decision is made by the Assessor; it is the final word. Be aware this could possibly cancel any decisions your loved one has made in the previous 6 months if they are now deemed incapable of doing so. Their decision is the Law.

Mom's Capacity Assessor was golden. This woman is also a medical doctor with a subspecialty in geriatrics, owns a clinic focused on cognitive legalities, *plus* her husband is a Judge. Wow! Can't get any better than that! So grateful for this legal advice. She was truly awesome.

Prepaying a funeral is a great idea. Tour different funeral homes, ask questions, explain what arrangements you want and get their fees. This process is much more relaxed and you will make a better informed choice for your loved one, if it's not done already. Compare prices. You don't need the stress of a last minute funeral arrangement. Always ask any funeral home if they're family run.

I found, family-owned funeral homes are far more flexible and accommodating in their fees and services. I found them to be the best choice for my mother's needs. Check them out before signing with a conglomeration.

Monies are held in trust. Once the contract is signed and paid for, the fees for the funeral services are set. There are no price increases. One less worry. It's a done deal.

The funeral home fees are separate from opening the plot and arranging for headstone/markers. Have this conversation with your loved one and respect their wishes. Call or visit cemeteries. Prepay for their services as well.

We all know funerals bring out the worst in people. Add nursing homes choices to that as well. Everyone is sensitive about these issues. Be prepared for the unexpected from friends and family. It happens to most people I've spoken with, and they didn't see it coming. So be prepared. If it doesn't happen – lucky you!

Open a **bank safety deposit box** in your name and place all the POA documents and Will inside. Otherwise anyone can remove and destroy it, especially if it's not in their favour.

PILLS, PSW AND THURSDAYS

I t has always been a fight to get mom to take her pills and these last 2 days were no exception. Her behavior tells me she's stopped taking them again, even though she says she has taken them. And I can't find any laying around.

The confrontation is always an obnoxious, verbal attack from her. She says I don't take care of her. I do nothing for her. She angrily demands "Where's my breakfast?! I'm sitting on the couch so why haven't you brought me my food?" She's told me that I'm living on easy street, to kiss her butt (not her words), I've got it lucky living in my room, she doesn't need any help, and she's not sick. It's just old age. It takes help from others to convince her to take her pills.

Accidental Martyr

Thankfully, the PSW's who care for her twice a week have a heart-to-heart discussion with her. I stay out of sight. It still takes some persuasion, but eventually mom takes her pills.

I wake her up in the morning for the Senior Centre's Thursday event. This outing involves socializing, games and lunch. Either my uncle or I have arranged to take her. We even confirm the arrangement the evening before. She agrees to go. However, she refuses to get out of bed in the morning and yells at me for trying to get her out of bed. She's adamant that she's always slept all day, even as a child. She's enjoying her dreams and doesn't want to get up. It's the same routine every Thursday. It is an event she has paid for in advance. She always has a nice time when she goes. It's getting her there that's the difficulty.

Eventually, we just stopped trying to take her. When she complains about sitting around the apartment, doing nothing, it's a conversation I avoid. It's not worth the stress. I've learned to pick my battles.

The PSW (Personal Support Worker) always phone to confirm their visit within one hour of arrival. Mom confirms the appointment. Then turns to me and asks who the PSW person is and why is she coming. She angrily denies she needs any help. It's a heated discussion about why she needs a PSW. Mention 'Dementia or Alzheimer's' to her and she yells at me that she doesn't have it, and she's fed up being told something's wrong with her.

I've learned she'll accept the PSW to come, if only to help her bathe and wash her hair.

Afterwards they can have a cup of tea together. Privately, the PSW tells me mom's complaining about me again. Apparently I do nothing, play on the computer all day, and that I go out all the time (of how I wish!).

She's also gotten out of bed looking for her ex-husband (who she divorced over 20 years ago) in the apartment. Another time when not feeling well she demanded I phone my dad to come over (he lives approximately 300 miles away.) Of course, I didn't bother him.

Then she actually called 911 again. I wasn't aware of this until the paramedics showed up at our door. This time I chose not to go over and sit with her in the hospital. I phoned the ER nurse asking that they call when all tests were done and I would come pick her up. They found nothing wrong with her.

Mom's mentioned these past 3 days of going into a nursing home. She thinks it's this apartment that makes her sleepy, that the building is too old. I had her repeat her comment and videotaped it for future reference.

I started using a crock pot to have a hot meal available for mom if I'm going to be out all day. That has worked well. I put a sign on the television, in large print, that her pills and juice are beside the couch as usual, and food is in the pot. She loves her particular yogurt, so I try not to let it run out. She eats one 500 litre container or two a day. Geriatrician at the hospital said to keep her eating it for the calcium. He wants the family doctor to inject mom with calcium, because mom just won't take all those pills. I've told the pharmacy to stop adding calcium pills in the blister pack because she refuses to swallow them. I had purchased chewable Vitamin C, D,'s and liquid calcium and iron. She takes that much easier, although it's still a battle.

I have become mom's personal assistant. I applied for a disability discount for mom's taxes and just got approval. So I have more forms to fill out for her. Always something to do on mom's behalf.

Oh yes, I'm encouraging mom to wear disposable underwear 24hrs because she doesn't make it to the washroom a lot, especially during the night. She has wet the bed, sheets and her comforter. In the middle of the night, I'd rather not be stripping and making her bed nor washing her. Am I being selfish? I don't think so.

I wouldn't normally divulge all this stuff, but I don't want family to think I do nothing all day, and nothing for mom. She wakes me up to have a conversation in the middle of the night. She cries like it's the first time when I'm forced to tell her someone she's trying to phone is deceased. The worst is when she asks why Steven (my recently deceased brother) hasn't phoned. That breaks my heart and we cry together. I have my own grief to work through, but now I realize, I also have hers.

LESSONS LEARNED:

Keep your family up-to-date on what's happening with your loved one right from the beginning. I appreciate you've got the right motive for doing this, and some of the accusations made against you are a lie, humiliating and a defamation of your character. You are too embarrassed to mention these comments to others for fear they won't believe you. However, family needs to know what's being said about you or done to you; even the problems you are experiencing. Ask for help. You are not alone in this. I have found this to be a common feeling among those who are family caregivers.

Stock the fridge with their favorite foods they can pick at. (Cheese, yogurt, fruit cold cuts, boiled eggs – you get the idea). Put these foods on a plate beside where they usually sit. I also have a little dish with nuts and another with candy on the side table, with a beverage. I found this helpful if I had to go out. When I returned I could see if she ate anything.

PSW's are your best friends. Get to know these people. They are aware of what you are experiencing and will work with you.

When the PSW arrives, leave. If you cannot, then stay away. Allow them to interact with your relative. Take the break. Let the PSW know where you are in case they need to ask you something.

Learn the signs that they're not taking their pills. Try to catch it early. After 2 days of not taking their dementia meds you're really dealing with Mom & AL at its worse. And it's not pretty.

Check out your community senior centers. They have all day events which includes lunch and social activities every day of the week. Mom happened to enjoy Thursday's events. Get their schedule and let your loved one choose a day. They can attend as many days as they wish, however there is a fee.

Take every opportunity you can (PSW visits, Senior Centers, hospital waiting time to name a few) to catch a break. Don't be a martyr. Plan these times for your own activities such as swimming, visiting friends; you get the idea. Take care of your own health be it mental, emotional or physical.

Just do it!

WHAT'S SHE SMOKING?

Mom runs (perhaps I'm exaggerating a bit) past my bedroom door heading to the living room with excitement written all over her face. She asks me "Where are my friends? What happened to the party?" She heard their voices and laughter clearly from her bedroom. She was so disappointed to realize she must have dreamt it.

The next day I could hear mom muttering and laughing in her bedroom. And she wasn't on the phone. I went in to make sure she was okay.

Yes, she said, she was talking. With who? I asked. With the man sitting on her window sill having a great conversation with her. We lived on the 6th floor of an apartment building. To have a man climb up and perch himself on the window sill was highly unlikely.

However, knowing my mom as well as I do, I checked the room for visitors. No visitors. We were alone. There wasn't any man. She had to be imagining it.

She knew he wasn't real. I asked if she was scared in any way. Not at all, she was having a nice time. Okay then, go back to your dreaming! Wish I could have dreams that kept me laughing!

I made an appointment to speak with mom's family doctor. Mom was getting difficult to get out of the house to go anywhere, even to her medical appointments. Mom has the walker, but can't walk far. She'll walk a bit, then feels weak and must sit down on the walker. So she ends up sitting in it, and I push her around the medical facility. I'm supporting her weight, helping to lift her up, drop her off and so on. It's exhausting.

So this time I went alone. The family doctor had a copy of moms Power Of Attorney on file, plus she knew me well from all the office visits I accompanied mom. Speaking about mom to the doctor was very productive.

LESSONS LEARNED:

Develop a good relationship with their medical doctors.

Make sure all medical doctors, government agency, and banks have a copy of the Power of Attorney (POA). Ask the bank to certify the documents, and get lots of copies. You will need them. Acting on behalf of your loved one requires a certified copy of the POA be given to every government ministry, each needing their own certified copy, as does organizations such as the banks and medical doctors.

As the dementia gets worse, Mom & AL will get worse in saying off-the-wall comments in public. Just be prepared for it. Haven't found anything that stops that from happening, so just go with the flow, change their focus and learn to laugh it off if possible.

Get a **Disability Parking Form** and bring it to their medical doctor to be filled out. So much easier getting around. To be able to park close to the entrance of buildings is really helpful, especially hospitals.

UNBELIEVABLE?
CRAZY? LIKELY TRUE

My friend Vivian went to visit her brother's grave site as was her weekly custom after work.

In the past, people have stolen the plastic flowers, wreaths off of the cemetery plot. It's unbelievable that people would do such a thing, but it does happen.

Imagine her shock when she walked towards her brother's grave to find the grass completed vanished from the plot! It was a perfect rectangle outline. The grass was MIA! She looked around at other sites, and no one had their grass removed. Everyone's grass was well groomed and beautifully green, as was her brother's grass last week.

She drove around the cemetery – everyone had their grass! Who steals grass? What was going on?!!! She immediately went into panic over-drive. Has someone very close to her died and she hadn't been told? OMG!

She drove up to the office to inquire what was going on. No, there wasn't any reason for grass to be removed. No, the grave was not going to be opened (the grass would be on the side if there would be). The cemetery personnel agreed to leave a note for the person in charge asking for them to contact Vivian with an explanation on Monday morning.

Panicking on her drive home, dreading how she was going to tell her parents that someone has stolen her brother's grass!! OMG! Desecrated his grave!!!! What the hell is going on!!!! Vivian's getting more nauseous as she's arriving closer to home. Her parents are not going to take this well. Wiping away the tears she approached her parents with the bad news.

Imagine her shock when they explained that they knew about the grass. In fact, they've paid someone to replace the grass two days ago. They forgot to tell Vivian. It was her fault for not asking before she went. Had she told them where she was going, they might have remembered and told her, maybe.

Her father has been diagnosed with early stages of dementia. Fortunately for him, he's lived in his house for over 40 years and knows where everything is without thinking about it.

Now when a crisis is apparently over, that's when you really crack up. It's when you can let your guard down; no one's feelings to protect. Vivian calls me and cries in her frustration. She lets the anger pour out about the stress this has caused her coupled with the grief concerning her beloved brother. Then, and only then did we start laughing! Yes, in her case she was dealing with Mom & AL and Dad & AL'!

If your relative's grass is the only one missing out of thousands of plots, rest assured, 'Mom & AL' was there!

LESSONS LEARNED:

If you can't figure out what's going on, it's because Mom & AL is creating it. If the problem or situation is way out in left field, bazaar, unbelievable and just doesn't make any sense; then you're dealing with dementia and not your loved one.

If you're pulling your hair out trying to solve a problem and not wanting to involve your loved one; stop. It's Mom & AL causing the problem! Go ahead and involve them! Hopefully you'll be able to understand what's happening. But don't count on it.

Stop pulling your hair out! The answer is simple. One mistake I hear everyone making when interacting with Mom & AL is that they try to reason with them. Reason isn't in Mom & AL's repertoire. They can't reason, just argue. They're really good at that. So don't engage in a logical conversation with Mom & AL trying to understand a problem.

Besides, they probably won't remember the situation anyway. And if they do, they'll deny any part of it. And let's face it, Mom & AL will say it's be your fault anyway!

Please, stop doubting yourself. You are not losing your mind – your loved one is! It's called dementia and it rears its ugly head at inopportune times.

Try not to takes these situations personally. Laugh it off, if you can. Talk to someone about it. Better to do that than get yourself into a full blown panic. Otherwise, you'll be the only one having a nervous breakdown. 'Mom & AL' will look at you and ask 'what's your problem?'

CAMERA....ACTION!

I came home to find a neighbor in our apartment with my mom. Apparently, they were outside enjoying the weather and had come inside for dinner. She kindly had made pancakes and brought them down for mom when she found mom lying on the floor and called 911.

I had arrived home just in time. The ambulance was coming to our door. I thanked the lady for all her help and she left.

I discovered mom had vomited all over herself and the floor. She was shaking like a leaf. She was in pain. It was horrible. She was having a heart attack!

The thought crossed my mind to take a picture of mom – crazy, I know. Perhaps the stress of the moment, but I doubt it. I resisted the urge.

The paramedics acted quickly and got mom stabilized and taken to the hospital. I stayed behind and cleaned up.

In the Emergency Department (ER), she had an EKG and other tests done. When I arrived, I found Mom was having fun with the two young, male paramedics. This was a definite sign she was feeling better (Apparently the paramedics must stay with the patient until they are moved to a bed.) Mom kept remarking on what great teeth the one young fellow had!

She was eventually given an ER bed and the paramedics left. As they were leaving, they said they never had such a great time with a patient! Mom had them laughing the entire time. She was flirting and teasing the young men.

Anyone who knew mom, knew she was just being herself. Even the family in the next 'room' were laughing along with them all! I knew mom was all right.

Once again, I thought of reaching for my cell phone to record this event. This time I did not resist. I knew mom wouldn't remember any of this tomorrow or the next day. And I would need proof. So I made the executive decision to document the event (video and photos).

I recorded mom explaining where she was and why she was there. I also took some photos of her in her hospital gown.

Mom was kept in the hospital for a couple of weeks. They felt she had had a small heart attack, with muscle damage at the back of the heart. When I visited her in the hospital she didn't know why she was there. Guess what? Yes, it was video time!

Later at home, she would argue that she never had a heart attack and would refuse to take her pills. After all, she said she would know if she had had a heart attack, right?

No argument here. Why? Once again it was video time! I gave her the ear plugs and asked her to watch the video on my cell phone. I left her alone to take it in.

This halted a lot of future arguments we would have. On video, she says she's had a heart attack and now feeling better. Mom was always shocked to hear herself explain what had happened to her. The proof was right in her hands. She was stating clearly that she had had a heart attack. Not me telling her. Nor anyone else. She couldn't argue with herself! And yes, she took her pills.

My only regret was not recording the paramedics. Mom would have enjoyed that!

LESSONS LEARNED:

Take a photo and a video with your cell phone. It's just handier. And when they challenge you, which is a guarantee they will, you have quick access to it. This was the smartest thing I ever did.

Also back up the photos and videos to your computer for safe keeping; I email them to myself.

Use the photos in your emails to keep friends and family updated. Keeping in mind your loved one's privacy and health.

When you video them ask questions such as "Where are you? How are you feeling? What happened?" Also mention the day and time for reference later.

PAGES MISSING

At 3:30 in the morning, mom called me into her room. She had felt her body weakening so she laid herself down on her bedroom floor, she told me. I helped her back into her bed and discussed, once again, the importance of using her walker.

She asked how long I was visiting her. She thought I had just come up for the night and was wondering how long I was staying. She didn't remember that she had asked me to move in with her because she was nervous about her falling. She didn't have the strength to lift herself up from the floor when she fell, or out of the bathtub.

She asked me if I've been caring for her and for how long. I told her 6 months I've been living with her, caring for her. I explained everything I was handling for her.

We talked for about an hour. We reminisced about her past. She wanted to know if her friends were still alive and how her family was doing. I was actually speaking with my Mom! She was wonderfully lucid!

I took this opportunity to explain to mom I was contemplating publishing my journal about caring for someone with dementia. It would be about our experience together. If it would help others, she gave her consent to move forward with the book. Besides, she always wanted a book written about her life growing up in Toronto, Ontario. This wasn't that, but close enough!

She told me she knew something was wrong with her mind. When she thinks of her past, parts of events are missing that she knows should be there. Her words were "my life is like a book with some pages missing". Such a perfect explanation of what dementia does to a person's brain from one who truly knew. I will always remember her words.

She also told me she couldn't visualize a thought or thing which was very unlike her since she was an artist. She thanked me for taking care of her. She told me she was very happy she had a daughter. She told me she loved me. We hugged and kissed good night.

I will cherish this moment. Mom was lucid. I was having a genuine conversation with my mom. It was loving and appreciative. 'AL' wasn't in the room. What a blessing.

LESSON LEARNED:

Cherish the good moments. They will be far and few between. I am so grateful I had this time with mom. In fact, journal moments like this. Otherwise the bad times will undoubtedly overshadow the good memories.

DEEZ PROBLEM?

M om's at home feeling weak and lethargic Saturday and Sunday, and by Monday she's staggering and throwing up. She's clammy and hot (she's never hot) so I once again called 911.

In the emergency department, you get to know the routine. You follow the same patients around the ER gauntlet. Wait for a bed, get in bed, get tests done, go get blood work and urine done, and wait for the MD. More tests? Finish? Oh goody! – "go wait in the waiting room" and they really do mean WAIT. We ended up sitting in the waiting room with a couple who were ahead of us in the testing process as well.

My mom has always been the type to talk to anyone who's around her. So why not this Baby Boomer couple sitting just two chairs away from us? Now don't think I'm not doing everything here to warn them! I'm discreetly leaning behind mom who's sitting in a wheelchair, mouthing the word "Alzheimer's" and pointing at mom! They nod understandingly. Mom engages this lovely couple. "Children?" "No." "Why not? Didn't want any?" "No, we didn't." "Was there a 'problem'?" They just smiled nicely back at mom.

Then without warning it happened. I should have seen this coming! Mom raises her hands in a double fisted position and wiggles only her baby fingers towards the husband, asking "Was it deez problem?!" smiling at them. Gratefully, they're laughing with me! Mom offers to take him down the hall to show him how she can help him correct the problem. Laughing, he says he's "too scared". "Well that's the problem then isn't it, you're just too scared!" We laughed for a long while. I think the levity broke some tension we were all experiencing in the ER. Way to go Mom!!

At this moment, the ER doctor comes over to us. I thought we were going to be told not to be so loud, but instead he says mom's looking piqued. "Has she lost any blood lately?"

I mentioned the staples in the scalp due to the ER fall last week. He looks at it and proudly states "Those are mine!" Fortunately, he arranges for mom to stay for 4 more days because her blood pressure keeps going up and down (perhaps causing some of her falls), and she's not eating a lot.

LESSONS LEARNED:

Record every important situation. This is the one, single, most useful thing I did. It made life so much better then, and still is useful today with mom in the nursing home.

On the video have them explain what's happening at that moment and give the date. So in the future, when she doubts your word, just play it back for her. My mom denied her mild heart attack ever happened. She refused to take her heart pills. I let her listen to the recording on my phone every morning around pill-taking time. It was the easiest method to convince her she had the attack (because after all, she's saying so) and needed the pills. I asked her questions in the ER, and she was explaining what had happened.

The Lesson Learned is that Mom & AL will stop arguing when they see and hear themselves talking. They will only believe themselves – not you, because you are the enemy. It also limited the amount of arguing we had. I showed her the appropriate video or photo, and it ended arguments.

Laugh. We have a choice to focus on the positive or negative side in every situation. Do your best not to take the situation so seriously or to heart. I will always have fond memories of this particular ER visit!

Cherish the moments when their positive personality is coming through. My mom has a great sense of Scottish humor. As you know, with dementia, they lose a lot of their personality and Dementia fills in the void. It's not pleasant.

WHERE HAS MY MEMORY GONE

L et's face it. How do you convince someone who's lost their memory, that they've lost their memory?

Discussions and arguments will never settle the question. Our loved one still has some memory. What they can't remember will depend on what part of the brain dementia has attacked. And this is part of the problem I was experiencing, especially in the beginning when dementia was undiagnosed.

My mom did remember some things, but not others. Which made me question what was going on with her. I knew something wasn't quite right. One minute she seemed her usual self, and then not. Later I had to rectify something she had done but she denied doing it. It was time consuming and a huge inconvenience.

That's when I began to take photos and videos of mom in any situation that she needed to be reminded of. When she fell and landed in the hospital (too numerous to count), I took pictures of her bruises, the stitches, any signs of obvious trauma so I could show her in the future. If she was waiting in the hospital Emergency Room for a bed, and she's in a hospital gown, I took pictures and videotaped talking with her about what had just happened. I'd lead with the questions and she'd respond.

This stopped most future arguments. It explained why she wasn't feeling well. Why she had headaches. Helped convince her to take her medications when she refused daily to take any of them.

When Mom & AL are stating facts, most likely it won't make any sense. You'll begin to try to understand what they said. Why did they say that? Why did they bad-mouth me to all her friends and relatives?

Here's another heads-up. STOP looking for reasonable explanations for what Mom & AL do and say. There are none. Logical, rationale explanations don't exist in Mom & AL's world. Stop beating yourself up.

LESSONS LEARNED:

Pick your battles and wait for the right time to proceed. This will save you a lot of grief and headaches.

Unless you're completely involved with someone with dementia, you cannot know what they put the caregiver through. It feels like Dante's Hell.

NEVER correct them. If you do, it will just snowball into a nastier, out of control argument. You'll end up being the loser. Trust me on this one! Mom & AL will take off the 'gloves' and go straight for your 'juggler'. This is inevitable. It will happen to you. They will push every 'button' you have. So save yourself the agony. Just agree with them. Or say "I don't know", "I have no idea", "You're probably right" and then quietly leave the room.

However, Mom & AL might follow you around trying to continue the fighting. Then change the subject completely. "Is it time for your favorite show? Have you heard from your friend? Would you like me to get them on the phone for you?" Distract them and they will move on.

WHO WAS MY HUSBAND?

I t was a nice Sunday afternoon. Mom was resting when the phone rang. A friend of the family informed her that her estranged husband with whom she had been separated for 8 years had died. If that wasn't bad enough, his daughters had already cremated him.

Mom cried tears of grief that turned into anger. My heart broke for her. I called her brother-in-law and they talked. He helped her feel better. I took this as a cue that I could leave and express my own grief.

It's Tuesday, or rather Wednesday at 2am. Mom wakes me up to sit down for a discussion. Luck was in my corner this time because she was somewhat lucid and wanted to know who her deceased husband was. Which one, since she had been married three times.

I reminded her of his name, what he did and where they lived. She couldn't remember marrying him. That scared her. She was cognizant that she knew him vaguely but couldn't locate the thoughts in her mind. She said it felt like there's an empty space in her mind where she couldn't pull out the information. She couldn't visualize. There were no photos in her mind. She was frustrated and upset.

So at 2:30 am until 4:30am, I was recapping her life with him, digging into her boxes to find photos to show to her of him, hoping to jog her memory.

I found photos of their beautiful bungalow in Niagara-on-the-Lake. The vineyard behind their backyard. Photos of how she had planned a birthday party for him there and rented a hall. He was so surprised she had done that for him.

One New Year's Eve, they celebrated at a local winery with a live band and dinner. No one else came to the event (weather was treacherous)! They had an entire band, dance floor and waiters at their beck and call. In the background were huge wine barrels. So romantic. They loved it.

While married, he had experienced a heart attack at home. Mom called 911. Had he been alone, she would have lost him. Mom, you're a hero! I could see the puzzlement on her face. She was trying hard to remember.

She remembered they were sweethearts when she was 17 years old. She vaguely knew she had stayed in touch with his family throughout her life due to the fact her girlfriend had married his brother, but couldn't remember any details.

When they rekindled their relationship, they had a lot of fun. He once lifted mom onto the hood of his car and starting kissing her. She was laughing so hard she almost peed herself! She was wearing this beautiful deep purple skirt and blouse. She looked gorgeous, so alive. They went into the Mandarin restaurant to meet up with his brother and sister-in-law trying to look respectable but they just kept laughing.

Mom really couldn't remember these events, although there was a hint that she should know this. Telling her not to worry, that today she might not remember, perhaps tomorrow she will.

She was angry at her disease and was venting. I held her close and we cried.

Throughout the next few weeks, mom needed to be reminded who had died. She was angry and frustrated that she couldn't remember him clearly.

Over the next several weeks she would repeatedly ask me who had died. Each time I told her, she experienced the same emotional grief over and over again, as if it was the first she heard the sad news. It was heartbreaking to watch.

This is such an ugly, insidious disease.

LESSONS LEARNED:

Remember they can feel that something is wrong with themselves but just can't pinpoint it. Their frustration level is so elevated.

It's not personal when they vent at you, although it definitely feels like it is. You just happen to be in the wrong place at the wrong time. Give them some space to vent. Don't try to correct them. Move on.

Sleep! It's the same rules as raising a baby. When the baby naps, you nap. It's a coping mechanism. So do the same with your loved one. When they nap, do the same. You have no idea when they'll wake you up in the middle of the night again.

I've noticed with dementia, persons have no concept of time. When the clock says 2 o'clock, there's no filter that distinguishes between day or night.

Use visual aids whenever possible. A picture tells a thousand words.

Have their preferred music playing, especially music from when they were young. It'll stimulate memories and put them in a good mood.

Take time out for yourself. You must rejuvenate otherwise you'll burnout. This is not negotiable.

A LITTLE RAIN MUST FALL

S o let me tell you about the rain that fell a week before I saw my rainbow. It was a hell of a rain storm!

Tuesday:

Mom's demanding to end the head pain. (She's had too many falls to count). She dials 911 for the ambulance and over she goes to the hospital with the paramedics.

I sat with her in the emergency department for what seem an eternity. The end result was a prescription for Tylenol #3. It's late. I walk over to our pharmacy next door to fill it but it's closed. I'm ashamed to say I cried walking home. How much can someone bear? I am exhausted. I wanted to be alone to cry and shut the world out.

Back at home, mom comes into my room and sits down opposite me. She tells me that looking after her isn't a life for me. "Put yourself first. Start dressing nice and go out". She leaves the room and returns minutes later, showing me that she is spitting as she speaks and then leaves again. I don't know if I'm coming or going, but one thing I do know for sure. I wish Mom & AL would leave, so I could have my mom back. I really miss her.

Wednesday:

Mom calls for me. I don't recall what the actual problem was this time. But whatever it was, in desperation I called my cousin for information about how to get mom into a nursing home. His mother, my mom's sister also has dementia and lives in a nursing home.

I started out our conversation, calm and collected. Then the more I explained my situation, the faster the tears poured down. I'm getting to feel so lost! He gave me great advice.

On a side note: Why when we cry does our nose clog up and mucus flows out of both nostrils? Isn't it bad enough our eyes are swelling up and tears are pouring down like a river? Then the situation is made more difficult because now one has to try to speak and breathe simultaneously because the nostrils are too busy creating and running a mucus factory. Do we never catch a break? Okay, thank you for allowing me to vent. Yes, I think I'm losing my mind.....back to my story.....

Thursday:

Mom calls me again for help to get up off the floor but this time she's shaking like a leaf. It reminded me of the mild heart attack she experienced previously. So I dialed 911 for the ambulance. This time Mom only had a bad sinus infection. I did the groceries while I waited for mom to be released. In our area, hospital emergency wait times are approximately 5 hours and longer.

Friday:

This day I walked into the living room to find mom laying on the floor with her head and neck up against the couch.

Although she weighs only 100 lbs., she's dead weight and I can't lift her. I try but she yells out about the pain in her neck. She has no strength in her legs to assist getting up, so once again I dialed 911.

I'm always concerned about the numerous falls to her head. So when in doubt, I'd rather paramedics help raise her.

Once again in the hospital ER tests results are normal. Apparently community health services had spoken to my mom without me present at the hospital. I requested to speak with the representative myself. I told them they were to speak to me with mom present. She has dementia and wouldn't remember anything discussed.

I had left a message for my uncle that mom was going to the hospital again. It was 7:45 am when the paramedics left with her.

During the previous night, I was lifting her up and helping her get to the bathroom. As I'm helping her back to her bed, once again she says this was no life for me. I told her not to worry.

Back at the hospital, my uncle joins us with perfect timing. Community health services sent an empathetic woman to discuss my request for a nursing home bed for mom. I explained that I was afraid mom was going to break her neck one day. I couldn't take care of her anymore. She told me there are no beds. I even offered to pay for a basic bed in the hospital until a nursing home became available. Sorry, no beds.

When all was said and done, we left. My uncle came back to the apartment with us. Fortunately, the mail arrived from community health services with the consent forms and nursing home choices. I filled the form out. My uncle reassures his sister that it was okay to sign it.

I left the two of them alone and I delivered the signed documents personally to the community health services. I'm crying hysterically while I'm driving over there. I am a mess! No one's lifting a finger to change mom's circumstance. The process takes so darn long!

Saturday:

Oh no, Mom & AL were in the room! We're on a roll this week!

Since Mother's Day until Nov 30 of this year, mom has been too tired or unsteady to get up and visit her great-grandchildren. She consistently declines to go for the drive with me. The drive also makes her nauseous and I often have to pull over so she can throw up.

This particular Saturday, after mom suffered with a fever and head pain which was treated with Tylenol and after multiply hospital visits, I made the mistake today of not inviting mom to join me for my weekly visit to see my grandchildren.

So this is what happened. My morning routine was to make her brunch and morning coffee. I turned the television on to her favorite channel. I placed a plate full of snacks, finger foods and fruit on the end table beside where she likes to sit. Great! Mom's good. Or at least I foolishly thought.

I had gotten dressed and was ready to leave. As I'm saying good bye to her reminding her again where I was going, she became furious with me. "This is no life lying on the couch watching television. Maybe I'd like to go!" She forgets about her head pain. Those Tylenol #3's are obviously working!

Yes, Mom & AL were back in the room. She became this unbelievably angry person yelling, screaming and threatening me right up close into my face. When she demands to talk with her brother Don, I was happy to comply. I tried phoning, but he wasn't home. I left a message for him to please call her and perhaps visit if he's in the area.

After all this commotion, I asked her once more if she wanted to come with me to see her great-grandchildren. She declined because she wasn't feeling up to it. UGH!!! Are you kidding me??!! What was the point of the angry behavior?

There's no logical explanation because I wasn't dealing with mom. It was Mom & AL. That was the problem. The amount of time, hours actually and energy expended getting mom settled so I could leave, then have Mom & AL turn on me, just sucked the life out of me! There's always some drama. Gratefully, being with my granddaughters gives me joy and a lot of laughter. Thank goodness I have my family!

Mom proudly claims she's now got a new personality which is much better than the one she had.

She also dictated that I couldn't take the car. Well, it's my car and so I left. After visiting my daughter, I returned home to find her sitting in the same place on the couch being pleasant.

Everything I've written for this past week is just the tip of the iceberg. I couldn't write everything down. It's too emotional and upsetting.

A lot of the verbal attacks just become my new normal. And frankly, I don't want to remember any of it. You try to let it slide off your back in order to survive.

I was trying to forget most of it because it just hurts so deeply. Sadly, I wasn't seeing any light at the end of the tunnel.

LESSONS LEARNED:

Mom & AL will become out of control. Dementia is nasty and will demoralize you. It also deprives you of a good night's sleep - every night. Keep in mind that sleep deprivation is used as a form of torture. Why? Because it works so well to break people! Get someone to cover for you while you get some uninterrupted sleep.

Taking on the care of my mother, I wish I had had a plan. I had no idea Mom & AL were so destructive and abusive. I would suggest my Ruler of Sanity to help you stay aware of how you're coping with your obligation. This will help you be proactive to take the appropriate steps long before caregiver burnout takes over you. You must commit to it.

I am at least happy I was able to keep my mom at home for as long as possible, and out of a long-term nursing home until it was absolutely necessary. On a side note, mom had to agree to enter into a nursing home. She could have said 'no'. I wish someone could have explained to me what the emotional and physical toll it would have on my health.

I realized as long as I was caring for my mom, the healthcare system wasn't going to put mom in a nursing home. She was not in crisis, and definitely not at the top of the waiting list for a nursing home. Besides, I was saving the healthcare a lot of money.

Once again, the following information is worth repeating and worth remembering: When nurses come to your loved one's home to assess their needs, be prepared. Walk your talk. If you feel like a mess then look like a mess! If you haven't slept properly, don't cover up the bags under your eyes! Case workers and nurses are not mind readers. They spend 30 minutes assessing the situation, which frankly isn't enough time to assess much. If you appear to be handling caregiving responsibilities effectively, you will receive in your home minimal help, if any. They will judge your appearance as to how you are coping. If you need help, act, talk and look like you need it. So walk your talk. This is not the time to go get a make-over.

THE NIGHT LIFE

Had my friend Millie stay over for the weekend with her little terrier.

In hindsight, my first mistake was having Millie sleep on the couch in the living room. I really should have known better.

Mom kept Millie up all night following the dog around the apartment. She'd also quietly approached Millie sleeping. Inches away from Millie's nose and declared, "Oh, you're not Kim. Do you want some tea?" They had tea. Time? Unknown but it was in the middle of the night.

Millie thought she could get sleep now but mom returned to the living room demanding Millie's pillow (Millie brought her own pillow) arguing that the pillow was hers.

Can you imagine this tug of war in the living room?! Her strength surprised Millie. Later still, mom woke Millie up to tell her jokingly, "Sorry we didn't get you a guy on short notice, but Kim and I are otherwise busy!"

Mom was having a fun time. This is my mom's sense of humor. I know she loved the dog being there. It would move from laying on mom's bed, and then jump off to return to Millie in the living room. Mom was just trailing the dog and keeping Millie awake!

I didn't know anything about what was going on between Millie and my mom. You never get a good sleep with dementia in the house.

I was catching some much needed sleep when Millie called my name, and out of bed I jumped. It was around 5 in the morning. Mom had fallen backwards, hitting the back of her head on the living room hardwood floor. I could cup my hand around the goose-egg. Millie called 911, Ontario's emergency telephone number.

Living across from the hospital, we waited to hear from the ER department before going over. We got the call that mom was fine and to come pick her up.

Back at home I made our breakfast and tea. Mom was happy watching television. So Millie and I decided to grab a coffee and park by the waterfront to recoup. Millie was especially exhausted! We stayed there for about an hour, then returned home.

On my apartment door, there was a yellow sticky note from a neighbor stating that mom had fallen (again!) and was taken to the emergency room.

Apparently mom banged her head outside while socializing with friends. This time she stepped backwards, tripped over the edge of the concrete sidewalk and fell on her head. The friends called 911.

So much for a weekend visit with a friend! I rushed over to ER after Millie went home. This was enough excitement for her. Millie couldn't believe what was involved caring for my mom 24/7 living with dementia. We've been friends for over 25 years, and she had never experienced anything like this.

Earlier in the week, when Millie and I were on the phone making our plans for this visit, mom came into my room to tell me off about something. Millie was shocked what she had heard.

She now had a better understanding of what I was living with. "Welcome to my normal" I said as we hugged good-bye.

With two falls in several hours, I requested she be kept overnight. The physician also wanted to arrange a team meeting for her long term care. Thankfully I agreed, and I went home.

I returned the next day to the ER to find mom in a different area with a nurse washing blood clots out of mom's hair! Mom wasn't bleeding when I left her last night! What's going on?

The nurse informed me that mom had a fall in the night. She asked me if I could comb mom's hair removing the blood clots. I am not a nurse or a support worker; nor did I work for the hospital! I didn't mind doing it, but what the heck? Good thing I'm okay with blood.

I asked a nurse taking mom's blood pressure if she knew what happened. She told me mom had fallen while walking down the emergency room hallway at night. The hospital never informed me of moms scalp staples or the fall. There were no messages on my cell or any calls on my mom's home phone. I wasn't happy to say the least.

As you know me by now, I took pictures of my mom. Pictures of her head staples, purple and black skin discoloration on her neck, head, arms, hands – all front and back. I documented everything that was relevant because I knew she wouldn't remember it.

They next moved my mom to another floor to keep her in. There was nothing more for me to do so I left to go home and bumped into my uncle coming to visit his sister. "You know you can't do this anymore, right?" I nodded in agreement. I obviously looked as bad as I felt. Really was comforting to know he cared.

Later I met with the hospital team before they discharged her. I found mom's disposable underwear was long overdue for a change. She had soaked her bed, the bed pad, sheets and her gown. When I helped her to stand up, her disposable underwear just dropped to the floor it was so heavy with urine. So I'm assuming she hadn't been washed either. She had been in there for a week. I complained and they took care of her needs. If you want something done right, do it yourself. Fortunately, I was taking her home.

Upon Mom's release, the doctor points out that mom has had over 5 visits to ER due to head injuries in 10 months. (Like this was news to me?!) "She *has* to use the walker" he says.

Well, let's consider the patient can we? Mom has eloquently stated that the "walker wasn't sexy". She's "not going to get a boyfriend using that!" I like her reasoning, but it didn't change anything. I could argue with her until I was blue in the face. Getting her to willingly use the walker was a lesson in futility. But that's another chapter!

LESSONS LEARNED:

Manage your time.

At the ER, ask the nurse for an approximate time before the MD sees your loved one. If it's going to be hours, try to get some rest and eat at home.

Also, if your loved one is taken by ambulance, it's also good to phone in to the nurse giving her details and ask how long before test results come back. You don't need to be there for 6 hours waiting in ER for test results.

Take this window of opportunity to sleep. Sleep deprivation is a form of torture. You can't function properly without a proper night's sleep.

Listen to your friends and family. For my uncle to comment that I couldn't look after mom anymore was more than just a head's up for me. It's a serious observation that you will soon burnout, if you're not already. Don't be a martyr. I really valued his input.

Keep up your association of close friends and family. Take the time to do something outside your caregiving hours, even creating dates with others who'll sit with your loved one so you can leave.

Never underestimate the strength of someone with dementia when they're angry or determined to follow through on something. A small, petite woman could overpower you if they put their mind to it. Their adrenaline must be spiking because they have the strength of Superman!

SELF-PRESERVATION
NOT OPTIONAL

E ver have the hair stand up on the back of your neck? I did.

Mom & AL came into my room one Sunday afternoon while I was working on the computer. She sat down on my couch angry, saying we can't live like this anymore. I was encroaching on her love life. She's lost men because of my living here. (She forgets of course, that she asked me to move in because she realized she was now much physically weaker and was having difficulties living alone.) This was just the polite stuff. It got really verbally nasty, to say the least.

As the hair stood up on the back of my neck, I thanked God I didn't leave my scissors out on the couch, because if I had, I was sure she would have stabbed me. This was a first for me with Mom & AL.

I didn't feel safe. I had to get out of here. So trying to change the subject, I calmly asked if she'd like to talk to her brother or my dad about her concerns. Yes to both. Her brother wasn't in, but I gratefully got my Dad on the phone. I explained to him that I had Mom & AL who wanted to talk to him. I needed his help.

As she talked on the phone, I grabbed my purse and drove down to my favorite spot by the water front to cry, think, whatever.

What did I ever do to deserve this? She knew all the buttons to push. And push she did. I wanted to die. Seriously die. I'm no drama queen but I assessed the lake. I could just keep walking out there until I drowned. Damn it! It looks too cold! Okay, so this is crazy talk. This is the spin-off from listening to Mom & AL. I don't want to die! I have 3 gorgeous, wonderful granddaughters with whom I want to be part of their lives. I also have two wonderful children! Reality check.

So I tried to relax to the sound of the waves by Lake Ontario but this time it just wasn't enough. I needed back-up. I called my friend, Vivian. I just let it all out, blubbering, sobbing all over my cell phone. I felt like a 7 year old having a meltdown! How could my mom treat me this way? The only suitable answer is that it's not mom. It's Alzheimer's. And I have to learn to separate the two. Besides…it's not personal. Yeah right, so why does it hurt so much? Because it IS personal.

Vivian invited me over, so I drove 30 minutes still crying without any thought as to why. The tears just flowed with a mind of its own. Vivian understood. We've known each other since we were kids. I didn't have to explain anything. I was safe. I could say anything and she understood. There was no judgement.

Afterwards, on my way home, I called another friend, who had a little dog. We got together and I played with her. She waged her tail and licked the tears off my face. I couldn't help but laugh. I chased her around the yard and had fun. I petted her, hugged her and walked her. It was soothing and medicinal.

I don't know what's happening to me, but I am always on the verge of crying now. In case you were thinking it, no, I am **not** PMSing!

Seven hours had passed by when I returned home emotionally exhausted, but ok.

Mom was watching television. "Oh, did you go out?"

Back home for more of the same….

LESSONS LEARNED:

Change the subject. Do not engage in any heated discussion/argument. Don't get sucked in. There is no solution. Distract them and they will move on.

You *must* have a mutual trusted friend or family member you can divert Mom & AL to. With my Dad, I would tell him Mom & AL wanted to talk to him. This was the 'head's up' for him to just to listen to her, don't argue. There's no point. She just needs to talk. He changes the topic to something she likes discussing, and she calms down.

Then **call a special friend** to vent. Choose someone who is sympathetic and has seen what you're going through. They must be 110% supportive and let you cry without any criticism. You will say things just to get the fear, pain, the hurt off your chest. This someone must understand, and allow you to vent without judgement.

Have somewhere safe to go to cry, scream, swear or yell, whatever. I would drive down to the waterfront and listen to the waves. Or drive to the far corner of a parking lot where you're alone to vent. Get a gym membership to smash some balls, swim the distance, run like your life depends on it because it does! Find somewhere that's 24 hours available.

If you don't have anyone, speak to a member of the Alzheimer's Society. The Alzheimer's Society understands the madness. It's the nasty side to caring for someone with Alzheimer's. Don't presume family will understand your circumstances.

Don't wait for a crisis to happen to take advantage of friends, activities and pets. Make it part of your week.

When the Personal Support Worker comes – leave! Even if for a drive with the windows down and with your favorite music blasting! Enjoy!

Take advantage of the opportunity not to be responsible. You deserve it. Treat yourself.

You know when the PSW is coming, so plan something for yourself. Be proactive.

ALZHEIMER'S SOCIETY MEETING

The room was full. Must have been 35 participants. Some were family members and others were friends supporting the caregiver.

You could pick the caregivers out of the crowd though. They looked exhausted, strained, bewildered, emotionally hurt, and no-doubt guilty for the way they were feeling. It was just like looking in a mirror.

Yes, they looked like they were hit by a moving truck. I knew the feeling, I knew the signs. They looked and felt just like me. Caregiving for a dementia sufferer takes its toll on the caregiver.

We took turns explaining our predicament and raised questions asking how to cope under such circumstances.

The room was full of people who totally understood where you were coming from and where you were heading. I felt safe.

One caregiver told the story of her husband believing he was back in WWII, and acting out survival strategies to hide from the enemy during the night. My heart broke for her. What a hell she was living through. And I thought I had it rough.

Now it was my turn to speak. I told the group that Alzheimer's has taken my mom. Mom, as I knew her was gone, but I had a reprieve because there were a few moments I would catch mom lucid. I intended to enjoy whatever good times I can before AL takes over completely.

I have some cherished moments with her I wouldn't have experienced had I not been taking care of her 24/7.

This was my sacrifice for the love of my mother. Would I do it again? Yes, but differently. More proactive with a support network in place.

LESSONS LEARNED:

You are NOT alone! Honestly!

Seek opportunities to confide in others who are caring for someone with dementia. There are large numbers of us out there. Don't be afraid to share.

When we've been beaten down by our loved one's dementia, like all types of abuse, you begin to doubt and question yourself. Try not to let that happen.

When you open up to a stranger who's also a family caregiver, you'll be amazed that they totally understand what you're going through.

I guarantee your conversation will help you both.

Go for it!

MIRACLES DO HAPPEN

Late September in a lucid moment, mom told me to not worry about her, that she'll "be okay. Go live your life. This was no way to live" not even for her.

After careful thought, I made the decision to move us to the other side of Toronto and gave notice we were leaving our apartment. My mom grew up in Toronto. I was looking with the intent of us moving together, but circumstances changed at a moment's notice.

Here it is....

Been a hellish week. I called an ambulance 4 times in the past 6 days. I would either find mom laying on the floor and I can't lift her up, or I won't lift her due to how her neck is situated.

And while in the emergency room at the hospital, I've requested and did meet with a community health service person about not taking mom home. I offered to pay for a bed in the hospital but was told firmly that there were no beds anywhere. I'm crying. I had already been in touch with them earlier about putting mom in a nursing home and nothing's happening. I just don't understand why nothing's being done. I'm afraid mom's going to break her neck, for crying out loud!

My hands were tied. Nothing I could do to change their minds. I felt so helpless, scared and exhausted. I took mom home once again.

Early this morning mom called me to help her. She had gotten herself pinned in and couldn't get up off the floor. She looked like a contortionist! She was soaked to the skin and had broken out in a sweat. When I tried to lift her up she would slip out of my hands. Yes, it's time for paramedics!

Our hospital is literally across the street. When the paramedics called the hospital ER department to say they were bringing mom in, they were told to take her to another hospital 30 minutes away.

It was upsetting to drive 30 minutes east for mom to get care, but I had no choice. The paramedics jokingly told me to bring a thick book as waiting times were long there too.

So I decided to stay home and wait for the nursing staff to call. I had lunch, did some housekeeping, gathered up something to read and off I went to the hospital once I received the call that tests were done.

When I arrived, I was shown into mom's room. The doctor came in to review her tests and he noticed an x-ray hadn't been done. He ordered it. He wasn't going to have a diagnosis until the result came back.

This might sound strange to you, but I had earlier taken a photo of my mom trying to shimmy her way out from where she had gotten pinned in. She was unsuccessfully trying to get up. So here in the emergency department I showed the photo to the doctor. He looked at it carefully, thanked me and said it was a great help in making his decision.

I sat beside mom while she laid in the bed waiting for results. She was sharing her view of the various shapes and colors, pictures and faces she was seeing on the ceiling and walls. None of it made any sense, of course, but this time I couldn't pretend to enjoy the show.

A nurse came in requesting a urine sample from mom, leaving some toilettes asking me to clean up after mom gave the sample. There was a chair in the room for such a purpose. Do you know the saying "the straw that broke my camel's back"? Well this was it for me.

I approached the nurse at her work station to tell her she'd have to help mom. I needed a break. "I just can't do this anymore" I said. "I'm going to sit in my car in the parking lot. Call me when the doctor returns."

I sat in my car for a while, then decided to go out for a drive and returned to the parking lot about an hour and a half later.

The nurse rang me and I returned to wait in mom's room. However, I arrived there, a male nurse was assisting mom with a walker going down the hallway to a washroom. Strange I thought, as the 'chair' was still in the room.

Soon the same doctor I spoke with earlier enters the room and shuts the door behind him. He points out the number of times my mom's visited the ER in just 6 months. Like I didn't know! "How are you coping with this?" he asks in his Australian accent.

The water works burst forth from my eyes like Niagara Falls! I was 'dumping' everything I've been doing for mom, her failing condition, ER visits and my difficulties getting her into a nursing home.

Oh my goodness! A professional was actually concerned about my mom! And Me! He got an ear full. Was I coherent? Who knows! Probably not; hysterical and desperate more likely.

This doctor kindly asked me how long had I been the 24/7 caregiver? Was I a nurse? A Personal Support Person? Any training at all? Did I have any support? (No, to all of the above). Have I spoken with my community health representative about getting mom in a home? What did they say?

At this point, as you can imagine I had a sudden attack of verbal diarrhea with no end in sight. (Pardon the pun!) "I was told there were no beds and there was a long waiting list. I even offered to pay for her to stay in a hospital for one night but was denied."

He told me what to do next time mom goes to the ER and what my rights were. Okay I thought, that was it. Mom's appointment was about to conclude.

This was the most helpful information I've ever received from any doctor or anyone else for that matter.

Imagine my shock when he said *I* was suffering from what's called caregiver burnout and that I couldn't do it any longer! OMG! I'm getting diagnosed as sick by the ER doctor - not my mother!!!

The doctor offered, if I wanted, to keep mom overnight. "Yes please, just give me one night's sleep!" Then he asked if I was mentally and emotionally ready to put mom into 'respite' aka an idle bed anywhere. "Yes, put her at the North Pole if need be, just keep her safe!"

But then the bigger, more outrageous thing happened. The doctor basically said 14 months of 24/7 care was just too long for one person to do, especially without any training. Although it was a lovely thing to do for my mom.

He said to me ever so kindly, "if you want her in a bed, tonight, I will make it happen. She won't be going home. And I am doing this for YOU!!!"

Oh silly doctor! I reminded him that our community health representative had already told me there *wasn't any beds*, anywhere, and just this past week! Money couldn't buy mom a bed! I know because I tried!

He told me there was another hospital 20 minutes north of us that had an available bed.

Now the floodgates of Niagara Falls transformed into Hurricane Kim! "What?!!! There is a bed??? I was told there were no beds!" His kind, helpful words whipped up Hurricane Kim into an internal frenzy. He leaned in to me and said "They ALWAYS SAY THERE ARE NO BEDS!"

For a momentary flash, I visualized myself tackling any community health representative I could get my hands on, wrestling them to the ground, beating their heads in for all the grief they've caused us. But then I'm not into fantasy. So back to reality. With Niagara Falls still rolling off my face (in fact, I barely notice it anymore), I gratefully accepted his offer.

As the doctor was leaving the room, the male nurse brought mom back in saying that the chosen hospital will take good care of her. The hospital team had already made the phone calls to find mom a bed to stay in until one opened up in a Long Term Nursing Home. Who would have thought I'd be the last to know. Everything taken care of. I was stunned, speechless, relieved and grateful.

Mom was now laying in her bed. I told her she wasn't going to be coming home anymore. There were just too many falls. The doctor has arranged for her stay at the hospital and she'll be getting physiotherapy during her stay. I explained that this same doctor had told me that I couldn't look after her anymore either, because my health has suffered. She said to me "I guess this is the time when it has to happen". I kissed her goodnight and left with Niagara Falls floodgates bursting forth. I'm sure people in the ER waiting room thought when I hurried passed them that someone had just died. In a sense it had.

When I got into my car, I called my dad. I'm telling him the good news but I'm still crying hysterically. He commended me for taking such good care of mom.

Next, I called my uncle. He was relieved that mom was now getting the care she needed, and that I could heal. There was no calming my tears. I just couldn't stop crying. Oddly enough, I found I needed to consciously breathe. I'm breathing quiet shallow.

I'm ecstatic to have had this medical doctor. He was heaven sent. What a blessing! I sent a thank-you card to this doctor, and another card of thanks to the emergency staff for their concern and efficiency.

LESSONS LEARNED:

As long as you're caring for a loved one at home and living with them, your chances of getting them moved into a Long Term Facility is next to never. If you're moving out, then that changes the situation into a crisis scenario.

It's your ER physician that makes the impossible possible, at least in my situation. A hospital emergency physician will place your loved one into a hospital bed to wait for a placement in a Home.

During mom's frequent ER visits, no medical professional in the ER noticed or even asked how I was coping.

Had I known what I do now, I would have acted sooner. I had no idea I could refuse to bring her home. I was always told 'no' and reluctantly accepted it.

I don't want anyone else to get emotionally and physically ill caring for someone we love.

You'll be the last person to realize you're burnt out.

And then you're no good to anyone, not even yourself.

ONE OF THE BIGGEST DECISIONS YOU'LL MAKE

I picked mom up at the hospital to drive her one-and-a-half hours to her new nursing home on the other side of the city on the edge of where I want to live and work.

The drive felt like it took forever. Even Mom commented on it. She had so many emotional questions for me while I drove. She cannot understand what was so difficult in my taking care of her. She can't understand why we just can't continue living together. It broke my heart. Why can't she go home to her apartment? Why can't she live alone?

To discuss this wasn't going to be productive, so I changed the subject. She would only be 20 min away from her great grandchildren who she adored.

Besides, this is only a temporary nursing home, not the 'forever after' place I told her.

I knew this place was old with a clinical feel to it. It had only one elevator but everyone waits patiently for their turn. Everyone willingly maneuvers to accommodate walkers and wheelchairs. No complaints from the staff that I could hear. It must be protocol for all nursing homes to have their staff be hyper-friendly to their clients. Everyone stopped and said hello or waved as they passed by. Besides they had an art class and I wanted mom in it. I hoped to rekindle mom's love of painting. She had lost interest in it.

We went to the 3rd floor. Although a basic rate, it was a semi. Mom got the bed closest to the door.

I noticed the top of the bedside table was dirty – so I cleaned it. I opened its drawers to find junk still in it; so again I used a tissue to clean it with hand sanitizer. There was obvious signs of not being cleaned on the floor. Okay, now it was time to complain. Housekeeping was notified and came a person came immediately to mop the floor and clean.

We were given plenty of apologies from upper management. The manager came to apologize to us personally. Apparently this floor experienced a few hospital emergencies. We were told that two individuals were in the last stages of life and were being monitored, with a prognosis of perhaps one or two day's life expectancy.

It was becoming obvious that this was not the floor for mom. I noted a keypad by the elevator. Some know the code, a staffer told us, but those with Alzheimer's were not given it because of the risk of wandering outside the premises.

Even with the code posted above the keypad, those with dementia were not able to understand the correlation and work the keypad. Welcome to the world on the dementia floor! I completely understand the need to protect the clients.

However, I wanted mom to be able to walk wherever she wants, on any floor in this building. No locked units for mom. When I initially toured this nursing home, I specifically questioned my tour guide about the locked units and ability to walk freely from floor to floor. Mom needed social interaction and the need to strengthen her leg muscles. She's to walk around as much as possible. Mom can hold a conversation and enjoys socializing. She definitely has dementia, but she's not out of her mind.

Mom and I took a walk around the hallway with the same intake person who met us initially in the foyer. She had the paperwork which I was to sign, but we'd take care of that after mom got to her room and settled.

Most persons were in wheelchairs and not cognitive, making weird vocal sounds. I was amazed at the numbers of them. Mom turned to me "Is this what I have been reduced to? Am I this far gone?" Then she saw my face,

"Why do you look unhappy?" "Cause, if I'm not happy, you're not staying here" I replied.

I pulled the Assistant aside explaining I wasn't going to put mom on this floor, and asked if there were any other beds available.

My mother, although diagnosed with Alzheimer's and Mixed Vascular Dementia, was in the 'present', could hold light conversation and was very sociable. I wasn't having her meandering around with her walker on a floor trying to talk with people who's (with all due respect) 'lights were on, but nobody was home'.

Another employee kept wanting to discuss the paperwork I needed to sign. I said I wasn't convinced I was letting mom stay.

It was originally arranged for me to join mom for lunch. Our arrival time was 11am. They said it would help mom with the transition. I agreed. Food was good and plentiful – one good sign.

I had joked that they should bring all the single guys together to meet mom. The Social Worker, in fact, brought us our lunch trays telling us there was good news. There was another bed on the fourth floor.

After lunch up I went to inspect it. Same bedroom two floors up. Brought mom up to see how she felt. This was so much better. Patients talking, waving, saying hello. We transferred all her clothes I brought for her move-in.

Of course the word was out by now about my lighthearted suggestion. Immediately one man was introduced to mom who was passing by.

Another in a wheelchair came over to introduce himself. Told his story why he was there and that he was the floor advocate, so if she had any problems, he would help her.

Mom was impressed. Nurses came in and introduced themselves. Mom's room was a busy beehive. She was content. We walked the floor. Some residents were in wheelchairs, some napping, others using their walkers. But most were talking to each other or at least saying hello. Things were looking up.

Arts & Craft's person, Bonnie, introduced herself to mom a second time. First was on the third floor hours ago. Mom and Bonnie continued discussing drawings, artists and crafts pointing out the Home's group artwork on the wall. Mom shakes her head "No, not interested. Painting. Oils. Acrylic. Water colors. Stenciling. But no crafts! Oh yes, lots and lots of dancing and music". "No problem, tomorrow there is an organ concert" she told mom and promised to fetch mom and take her down.

I reminded mom this was not where she was going to stay forever. (Little did I know). It was temporary. It was just the first bed that came up now that she was to be discharged from the hospital. She was okay with that.

Took an hour to discuss and sign the paperwork and write a cheque. Then I was handed over to the nurse in the family room, a very small room off a small corridor. As the nurse was asking me for mom's medical history, I could hear the social worker talking on the phone in her office.

She should have spoken quieter and with the door closed tightly to respect patient confidentiality, but she didn't. I could hear her relate my complaint about the room not being cleaned, unhappy with the floor residents and everything else I had said.

But I almost died when she mentioned 'she wanted single men brought to her'!!! I stopped my conversation with the nurse. "Who's that talking?" I asked in shock. "Sally, why?" "Well, she's discussing my mother, and no, we didn't seriously ask for single men to be brought to mom's room. Call her in here."

She did some back peddling when I approached the subject. "No, no, we like to mention things like that to each other". After our discussion, I hope she learned some valuable lessons here. I certainly did. I had joked during lunchtime that staff should bring all the single guys to meet mom. Mom and I were laughing as I said it. However, I was taken seriously, and that wasn't my intention. I was just joking! Although, mom did enjoy the attention from staff and fellow patients.

Mom and I were both very tired by now. She laid down on her new bed facing away from me towards the window. I leaned over while sitting in the chair that was beside the bed, crumpled my coat against her and put my head down beside her. She reached behind her and kept her hand on the back on my head. Mom told me it felt so comfortable. I agreed. We must have slept for 15 min just like that. I felt like her little girl again receiving affection from mom. I am grateful for this moment. It was tender. It was loving and kind. It was a rare moment between us, considering all that we've gone through. I was once again sharing a nice moment with my mom, and Mom & AL wasn't in the room.

A bell had rung announcing dinner time. I helped mom sit at her designated dinner table. I read her the menu choices hung on the wall. She chose ginger chicken. A good choice I thought. I waited for the food to arrive. Amongst the commotion I kissed mom good bye and left. Timing was right to say good-bye.

Got in the car feeling numb. I reasoned that I knew she's there for her safety. I know this decision is right. I know medically it needs to be done for her sake, but also because my health has suffered. I know I need to live my life, a life which I am devoid of. It's all in the process of living our lives. This makes common sense. Medical sense. A 'must do'.

All the logical, reasonable answers I came up were sound and rationale. I couldn't handle mom's health needs any longer. I did my best, but now it was not enough. It was time to leave her care with qualified people.

But it still really, really broke my heart. No one prepares you for this.

Upon arriving home, as I walked out of our apartment elevator, I felt the loss. It was the same loss I felt when my older brother passed away a few years previously. There's this void. An emptiness. The realization that I wouldn't be saying good night to mom when I turn off the lights tonight. I wouldn't be giving her a hug and kiss good-night as I tucked her in. I burst into tears and just let them flow. I am so damn exhausted on so many levels.

LESSONS LEARNED:

Home Choices: Know ahead of time what you'll do if you didn't want to leave your loved one at one of your choices.

As long as it's not your first choice of a Nursing Home, your loved one stays on the roster for the #1 choice. If you're bringing her from a hospital to a Home, definitely ask the question. I didn't know whether I could return my mom to the hospital after she was discharged. It would have been good to know. At this particular Home they had art lessons and an art room. I felt with mom being an artist it would something she'd enjoy doing.

Doing the right thing isn't easy. And frankly, no one said it would be. It will be, on one hand heart-crushing. On the other hand, a huge weight off of your shoulders. And when I say 'weight', I really mean it. It really felt like an unbearable 150 pounds was lifted off me. That's the stress, strain, exhaustion, anger, frustration, grief and abuse finally being released.

Freedom. And it feels odd, even uncomfortable because it's been so long since you've had any of it.

Accept it.

Welcome it.

NO REGRETS

D o I feel guilty allowing mom to go into a nursing home? Initially, absolutely. When I first left her there I cried my eyes out driving home. (OMG will I ever stop crying!!)

When I got past the negative emotion and started to focus on the positive, I began to feel a sense of relief. Mom was safe.

Nurses made sure she took her medications – a fight I had daily with mom, and did not always win either! She was now eating regular meals and snacks. Mom was putting on a few pounds. Nurses assisted her when she fell. No one called me in the middle of the night. What a blessing for both of us.

Now comes the time to sort through her belongings. She had told me previously what she wanted done. Who was to get what, and I made sure I respected her wishes.

The gut-wrenching problem was that this felt like a death. This is what you do when someone dies. It's tough to say the least.

Mom had 82 years of memories stored in her apartment. It was overwhelming for me. Thankfully mom was still alive and I could still visit her. I counted my blessings.

Now that she's in a nursing home, I've noticed she doesn't remember visits, telephone calls, special occasions, or conversations.

I show her photos and videos from my laptop. When I was sorting through her photos when I was cleaning out her apartment, I took pictures of them using my cell phone and uploaded to my laptop. Now when I visit her, I let her watch family and youthful photos of herself play for hours for her.

She enjoys seeing them and remembers some details, especially the older ones. She gets excited when she remembers the event and talks about what's happening in her photographs.

Sadly, she doesn't remember her paintings she did over the years. They are beautiful. I had two portraits hanging in her room to remind her that she did these works of art. I would find them taken down when I would visit. She said she thought she was bragging.

LESSON LEARNED:

No one wants to place their loved one in a home, but the time does come when you don't have a choice. Accept it gracefully. It's in everyone's best interest.

ALL IS NOT WELL

I n the first few months on the fourth floor, mom had found herself two boyfriends. She was excited, obviously happy and smiling. Gees, if I had two boyfriends I'd be happy too! When I was leaving the nursing home, she happily wave me good-bye. Inside I cheered 'way to go Mom'!

Happiness, however, didn't last too long. Mom was now crying to me that the nurses were breaking it up. When they were holding hands, the nurses would tap their hands apart telling them not to do this.

The nurses didn't call me about any of this until one day they caught mom sitting on her boyfriend's lap in his wheelchair.

I laughed when they told me about it. I could visualize my mom sitting on his lap with their arms around each

125

other with big smiles on their faces. Unfortunately, the nurses didn't share my joy. And the nursing home wasn't having any of it.

Their solution to this problem was to move her to another floor. I understand the legal concerns for someone with dementia being taken advantage of, and possible family concerns. But as far as I was concerned, as long as mom wasn't going to get pregnant, was over the age of twenty-one and the guy didn't have a wife; leave her alone. And I told them that.

Just because a person is a senior and has dementia, doesn't mean they don't want companionship. They are still human, with natural feelings enjoying the warmth of another person. Holding hands. Hugging. Smiling. Flirting. The feeling of being alive and wanted. We ALL need that regardless of age. Emotions don't get switched off because we're in our twilight years.

So anyway, mom gets moved to the fifth floor now. Thankfully, mom was making new friends, walking everywhere. Her strength in her legs has improved dramatically. She was taking the elevator and visiting others on different floors. She was happy. I was thrilled.

Apparently, mom was also twice found outside the nursing home waiting by the front entrance. When asked what she was doing there, mom said she was waiting for her brother to pick her up to visit her sister. This, of course, wasn't true.

Then again on another occasion, I received a call from the Home asking me to speak to Mom. Sure thing. Mom anxiously tells me that she's just visiting friends at the Home, but that they mistakenly believe that she lives there and won't let her leave! She was so upset. I asked mom to look at the bracelet on her wrist and to read it to me. She read her name and the name of the nursing home. I told her she did live there and she was home.

Finally the last straw. I received a phone call that Mom was found in the basement which was off-limits because that's where the laundry room and kitchen were located.

It didn't matter. Mom had gone AWOL too many times and now this. The nurse told me that they wanted mom on the secure dementia floor which originally I had refused to put her on. They didn't have enough staff to follow mom around they explained. They didn't have enough staff to watch who comes and goes down the elevator.

And the main floor, front receptionist? That wasn't their job either to watch who leaves the building. Besides, someone wasn't always at the Front Reception. (Something to keep in mind when you're touring nursing homes to make your choices.)

I was emphatically told it was my responsibility if any harm comes to my mom, not theirs if I refused to move mom. The nursing home was located extremely close to a very busy highway. What choice did I have? I had no leg to stand on now. I had to consent reluctantly. I was made to believe my hands were tied.

The second floor had a form of security. Meaning? You had to be able to read the directions posted over the keypad outside the elevator to leave the floor. I disliked this floor and it bothered me visiting her there. The residents were basically non-verbal. No, let me correct that; they were not conversational.

It's the floor where you hear others crying out loud (screaming more like it). Those in wheelchairs were lined up along the corridor walls. Their heads were hanging over to the side. They used their voices, but only indistinct sounds came out.

This is where my mom, a woman walking around making friends, having conversations with others, joining in activities, becoming stronger each day by walking everywhere, was now stuck. I called it Lock Down.

On most occasions when I visited mon I now found her lying on her bed. She'd tell me the woman with whom she shared a room was crazy and conversations never made any sense. And last but not least, 'Get me out of here'.

She kept accusing me of putting her in the Home. I would tell her the doctor made that decision, not me. I showed her photos of her injuries so that she would hopefully understand why I couldn't look after her anymore. I showed her the video where she said she wanted to go into a home.

But this floor was zapping my mom of life. I could see it, but didn't know what else I could do. I asked for her art therapy classes to continue, but the Home had run out of funds for their fiscal year. Perhaps next year.

My mom deteriorated very quickly. She couldn't walk more than ten steps without falling. Even using her walker she would feel the need to drop to the floor. They put mom in a loaner wheelchair. I was visibly agitated about this telling the nurse if I ever found my mother parked in a wheelchair in the hallway like the others, there would be hell to pay and I would be taking her home with me.

I did have mom on a waiting list for other Homes, but it seemed like it takes forever to get her into one of my top 3 choices. In fact, it does take forever to move them unless you can afford a single room at a very high price.

BLOWN OUT OF THE WATER

Trust me, I never saw it coming.

One Saturday in April, I took mom for a day's outing. Our routine would be to get her hair cut, visit friends and then have her get a pedicure and manicure. On our way home, we would stop in to see my grandchildren, mom's great-grandchildren. Always a fun time.

At the nail salon, my eyes and jaw fell to the floor in horror. I was trying to remove mom's socks when I felt some hard bar stretching across the end of her toes making it impossible to remove her socks. "What was the nursing home placing in her socks?" I asked myself. I rolled her socks off beginning with her ankles and held onto the bar by her toes.

Unbelievably, her nails had grown to the tip of her shoes, then made a dramatic turn to the left (or right depending on the foot) and was growing on top of the next toenail!!! Her nails were hard, thick and shaped like an allen-wrench, like the letter 'L' laying sideways on her toes. They formed a hard, solid, interlocking bar. I was in shock.

Obviously, she had no nail care since I last took her for a pedicure 6 months ago. Mom was listed as a diabetic. She should have received regular diabetic foot care as a matter of course at the Home.

And how does this not get noticed by staff when dressing and undressing her morning and night? Or when being bathed twice a week??!!

(By now you know me, yes I took a picture of her nails with my cell phone. I can visualize myself taking the photo, but do you think I could find it later? No!! To this day I have no idea where those pictures went. I'm so angry!)

Moments later, the woman who appeared to own the nail establishment seated herself in front of mom's feet to perform the pedicure. I'll never forget the look on her face, nor the broken English she loudly spewed at me. "Tooooooo long! You wait toooooooo long! No good! Free months, free months!"

I was humiliated in front of all these customers and people working in the store. I tried to explain my horror that this was the first time I've seen this and that I was more shocked than she was.

The only mature thing I could do was say I'd be back in half an hour. And that I was going next door in case she needed me. There, I bought a delicious slice of Rum cake and drank two heavenly cups of coffee. Yes, I was self-medicating.

That evening when I returned mom to the Home, I complained to the nurse on staff. Then on Monday morning I complained to the Director of Care about her toenails as well as her cognitive decline. She showed concern and offered to move mom to the fifth floor if I wanted. If I wanted? Are you kidding me? I was told I didn't have any choice in the matter when she was placed there about eight months ago! I hated the second floor! Move her to another floor? Hell Yes!

That move was done in a matter of a day. I returned to make sure everything of hers was moved over to the fifth floor. It wasn't. So I notified the nursing station. I was waiting for someone to go down and retrieve her things left behind in a cupboard. A day went by and it still wasn't done.

So I went to the floor myself asking a healthcare person to accompany me. I took mom's box of things to her room and put it away.

A meeting was scheduled with mom's entire health team including the Director of Care. They offered their apologies once again, thanking me for giving them a second chance. They asked how they could help my mother.

So I told them. If she gets a boyfriend *leave her alone*! Get her walking around, if it was now physically possible. (They will tell you that it's part of the disease that they start falling; and perhaps it's true, but my mom changed drastically in a negative way, too quickly on that floor to blame Alzheimer's totally).

I was reassured corrective action had been taken on the second floor regarding mom's lack of care, but due to confidentiality the Director of Patient Care couldn't tell me what was done.

I told them that floor had sucked the life out of my mother. I started crying in frustration and anger as I'm demanding what better be done for my mother. They were very concerned, cooperative and empathic. Too little too late.

LESSONS LEARNED:

Know your loved one's rights. It's posted usually near the entrance area or by the elevator.

There's a confidential telephone number listed there to call to complain about nursing home care. When in doubt, call it. You will be given a reference number.

I only reported this incident after a friend, a retired nurse told me that the toenail problem falls under neglect, and that I should report it. After all, I no longer any proof.

So don't procrastinate. At least the neglect is documented. I spoke to the Ministry about mom's situation and received a reference number. However, it took well over a year for someone to contact me that an unscheduled Home visit will take place to investigate my complaint. At this time I added everything else that I was not happy with.

Stay on top of their care. Don't presume everything's alright. And for heaven's sake, check their toenails.

Remember, the 'squeaky wheel gets the oil'. Be proactive.

Make yourself known to the staff and visit on different days of the week and at different times. Not that it would have made any difference in mom's case. Keep everyone on their toes. Oops, pardon the pun!

Go to the Director of Care for any problem. They make changes happen. I wouldn't bother with the nurses on the floor. They're only doing what they're told to do.

Talk to the Social Worker at the Home about any concerns as well, such as companionship issues.

Although mom was still on the Long Term Care Homes Choice List, she was no longer in crisis, and therefore, her placement to actually get into my preferred home was not happening.

Remember that when you create your choice list. If one Home is just 'okay', realize it might be their 'forever home' unless some criteria makes it necessary to move them. So think twice about putting that Home on your List.

When taking photos on your cell phone, email them to yourself for safe keeping. Wish I had!

P.S.

It took about a year to hear back from the Ministry that they were finally going in to check out the Home. I thought, why bother now? I mean, we're talking about toe nails here. I didn't expect any satisfaction at this point, but I was wrong.

Just received a phone call that they had investigated my concern and they found some problems during their investigation which were going to be posted on the Ministry's website that reports any problems they find during the unannounced investigation.

They offered me my own personal report which I look forward to getting in approximately three months' time.

A NEW BEGINNING

The nursing home called me in for a meeting with mom's caregiving team. Apparently within a 20 day period mom had tried to 'escape' her floor 30 times. They would try to get her out of the elevator and mom would fight them off. Everything was documented.

The intent of the meeting was to notify me that they could not guarantee mom's safety if she escaped. They didn't have the manpower or the funds. They were moving staff around to walk mom around to keep her busy and giving her a sleeping pill in the mid-afternoon to get her to sleep earlier. Yes, mom was always a night owl.

I agreed I wanted mom moved and have been trying since the nail incident, without success. So how could they move mountains?

They arranged for me to work with their Social Worker who called various homes (I already had a list made up) that had the necessary security measures in place. Such as bracelets that buzz the door if they get too near to the exit, or lock the door so they can't get outside unassisted. Everything was put in place. All I had to do now was wait.

I explained to mom what was happening. I gave her two thumbs up, a hug and a kiss for her escaping attempts! I told her it's because of her behavior that she's getting out of here. Everything I was doing by the rules, wasn't achieving anything. Way to go mom!

When I got the call that a bed was available (it took a few months), I knew I had to move quickly. I asked if the Home would pack up mom's belongings, which they did. When I arrived there I double checked that everything was packed up and out of her room, loaded the car and then finally drove mom across the city.

On behalf of mom, I bought a bouquet of roses for the staff on mom's floor, and a separate bouquet for the art & entertainment therapist who was always so nice to mom. They were all so delighted to receive the flowers.

When I arrived at the new Home, they were very accommodating helping me unload my car and wheeling mom's things on a cart. The room mom is in is lovely.

It's a basic room in a new facility, which means she has her own large space divided by walls with a curtain acting as a door. She shares a huge washroom with another lady with a large oval mirror over a pedestal sink with full cupboards on either side assigned to each woman.

Mom has an enormous window that looks out over the backyard and a walkway used by cyclists and joggers. It's bright and cheery. A wing back chair sits beside the window.

There's a small café in the front foyer with comfortable seating where mom and I sit enjoying chocolates and cappuccinos sitting near the large fish tank. She enjoys watching people. She remarks that she knows all these people which she doesn't, but who cares. I just smile and nod in agreement.

There are two large outside gardens on her floor which I take her out into to enjoy the scenery and get fresh air.

I can relax now.

It's wonderful.

www.ingramcontent.com/pod-product-compliance
Lightning Source LLC
Chambersburg PA
CBHW070932210326
41520CB00021B/6905